SURFACE IMAGINATIONS

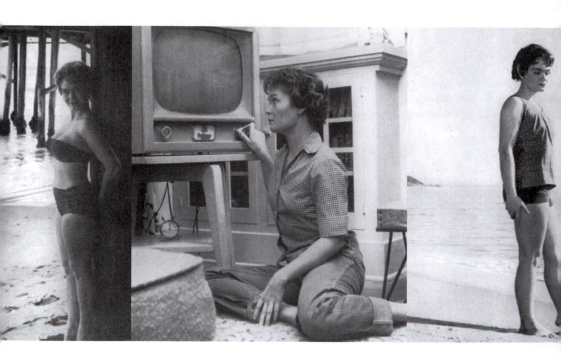

SURFACE

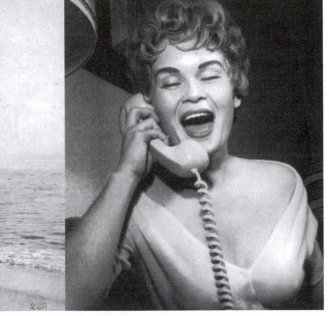

IMAGINATIONS

Cosmetic Surgery, Photography, and Skin

Rachel Alpha Johnston Hurst

McGill-Queen's University Press

Montreal & Kingston · London · Chicago

ISBN 978-0-7735-4600-4 (cloth)
ISBN 978-0-7735-9774-7 (ePDF)
ISBN 978-0-7735-9775-4 (ePUB)

Legal deposit fourth quarter 2015
Bibliothèque nationale du Québec

Printed in Canada on acid-free paper

This book has been published with the help of a grant from the Canadian Federation for the Humanities and Social Sciences, through the Awards to Scholarly Publications Program, using funds provided by the Social Sciences and Humanities Research Council of Canada.

McGill-Queen's University Press acknowledges the support of the Canada Council for the Arts for our publishing program. We also acknowledge the financial support of the Government of Canada through the Canada Book Fund for our publishing activities.

Library and Archives Canada Cataloguing in Publication

Hurst, Rachel Alpha Johnston, 1977–, author
Surface imaginations : cosmetic surgery, photography,
and skin / Rachel Alpha Johnston Hurst.

Includes bibliographical references and index.
Issued in print and electronic formats.
ISBN 978-0-7735-4600-4 (bound).–ISBN 978-0-7735-9774-7 (ePDF).–
ISBN 978-0-7735-9775-4 (ePUB)

1. Surgery, Plastic–Psychological aspects. 2. Photography–
Psychological aspects. 3. Skin–Psychological aspects. 4. Beauty,
Personal–Psychological aspects. 5. Body image. 6. Self-esteem.
7. Self-perception. I. Title.

RD119.H87 2015   617.9'52   C2015-904925-3
                                      C2015-904926-1

CONTENTS

FIGURES

ACKNOWLEDGMENTS

Without the generosity of spirit demonstrated by the seven women whose narratives of cosmetic surgery shaped my understanding of the experience and industry, this book would look very different. To Diana, Leah, Melinda, Nicanor, Tigerlily, Tonya, Victoria: thank you. For most of us, I think, it is difficult to live comfortably in our bodies – this is even more so for those of us whose bodies are shaped by genealogies of racism, sexism, classism, homophobia, transphobia, ableism, and sizeism. Even more difficult, however, is putting this complexity into narrative. I admire your courage in sharing a part of your history of embodiment with a stranger in order to help better understand how cosmetic surgery addresses – and does not address – how hard it is to live in a body.

Kyla Madden, senior editor at McGill-Queen's University Press, has been an extraordinary support. When we began working together on this book, the work had been a major part of my life for several years and I was eager to get it published and out of my life as quickly as possible. However, Kyla pushed me – calmly, firmly, and gently – to continue the work to make it better. Never have I received such thoughtful and precise feedback. It was thrilling to work with someone so skilled at recognizing, and then explaining, what my work could become. Thank you, Kyla. Indeed, I am grateful to all the staff at McGill-Queen's University Press who assisted with the production of this book. I am indebted to the anonymous reviewers, whose feedback generated new lines of thought and strengthened the arc of the book. Thank you for supporting my work and helping me refine it. I received invaluable assistance from librarians and archivists in tracking down and reproducing images: Lise Brin, St Francis Xavier University; Philip Skroska, Bernard Becker Medical Library, Washington University School of Medicine; and Mindy Tuana, Gerstein Library, University of Toronto. Thanks to Kate Merriman for carefully copyediting my manuscript, and saving me from future embarrassment! And last but not least, thank you to Mary Newberry for preparing another excellent index and for her keen eye for detail. Of course, any errors and infelicities are my own.

The Associate Vice-President of Research and Graduate Studies at St Francis Xavier University and the St Francis Xavier University Council for Research provided research funding to support the publication of this book, for which I am very grateful. This book has been published with the assistance of a grant from the Federation for the Humanities and Social Sciences, through the Awards to Scholarly Publications Program, using funds provided by the Social Sciences and Humanities Research Council of Canada.

Earlier versions of sections of this book were published in articles and book chapters, and I am thankful for permission to reproduce them here. Specifically, the poetic transcription "Grandmother and Mother" appeared in "Negotiating Femininity with and through Mother-Daughter and Patient-Surgeon Relationships in Cosmetic Surgery Narratives" in *Women's Studies International Forum* 35, no. 6 (2012) and is reproduced with permission of Elsevier. Parts of chapter 2 appeared in the following articles and book chapter: "Complicated Conversations between Interviewing and Psychoanalytic Theory" in *Reconstruction* 9, no. 1 (2009), reproduced with permission of *Reconstruction*; "Surgical Stories, Gendered Telling: Cosmetic Surgery through the Perspectives of Patients and Surgeons" in *Gendered Scripts in Medicine and Narrative*, edited by Angela Laflen and Marcelline Block and reproduced with the permission of Cambridge Scholars Publishing; and "Happiness and Its Discontents in the Cosmetic Surgery Photograph," in *Topia: Canadian Journal of Cultural Studies* 25 (2011), www.yorku.ca/topia. And finally, a section of chapter 4 appeared in "The Skin-Textile in Cosmetic Surgery," in *Skin, Culture and Psychoanalysis*, edited by Sheila Cavanagh, Angela Failler, and Rachel Hurst, 2013 and is reproduced with permission of Palgrave Macmillan.

I am grateful for the many friends, teachers, and colleagues at St Francis Xavier University (where I am currently a faculty member) and York University (where I completed graduate work) whose paths have intersected with mine in the past or present. Many have provided intellectual and/or emotional support for this work through close readings, celebrating my successes, sharing food and ideas, or inspiring me to keep going. Thank you to Paola Bohórquez, Deborah Britzman, Sheila Cavanagh, Shana Calixte, Angela Failler, Susan Ehrlich, Clare Fawcett, Nancy Forestell, Celia Haig-Brown, Krista Johnston, Marlene Kadar, Kristine Klement,

Deborah MacPhail, Jennifer Musial, Gail Vanstone, Charlene Weaving, and Melissa White, in particular.

I love and am filled with gratitude for my family of origin and my chosen family. Thank you to Marjorie Hurst, my mother, and George Hurst, my father. This book is dedicated to you, to honour my Mom in the present and in loving memory of my Dad. I am grateful for the support of my best friend and little sister Stefanie Hurst, my sister Kim-Ellen Hurst, and their families. Finally, thank you to my loving friends Ryan Billington, Megan Bulloch, Maria Gentle, Sabina Hikel, Stephanie Johnston, Sara Mackenzie, Michael Newton, Noël Patten, Shawn Thomson, and Baharak Yousefi.

Surgical Culture Transformations

DISCOVER MY FACE/DON'T HESITATE CLICK ON ME![1] This excla-
mation and command once appeared on the front page of French performance artist ORLAN'S website, beneath her name. And, indeed, as I
navigated my cursor over her face, her face transmogrified into a map of
links to various pages on the site featuring images of her artwork; up-
coming, current, and past exhibitions; her writing; review essays about
her art; and other materials related to her work. ORLAN'S face maps an
assortment of eclectic cultural referents; it is a discoverable face that is
strangely beautiful, although not according to the standards exemplified
in North American fashion magazines. Her hair is wild, half of it grey-
black and the other half white: it rises into the sky, an evocation of the
Bride of Frankenstein. Hazel eyes gaze out from round, black plastic
glasses with thick yellow arms, frames reminiscent of Sigmund Freud's
iconic glasses. ORLAN'S dark red lipsticked lips purse together in a not-
quite smile, a hybrid of vampy film noir actresses like Veronica Lake and
the art history icon Mona Lisa. Her temples jut out, augmented with silicone implants originally designed to enhance cheekbones; for this facial
feature, we have no immediate cultural referent. When ORLAN spoke at
the Ontario College of Art and Design in the fall of 2008, she had made
up her otherworldly temples with luminescent glitter that fascinated my
gaze throughout the talk. These temples, made of silicone and highlighted
with pearlescent makeup, gleamed. They had been implanted during one
of her cosmetic surgery performances from the series "The Reincarnation
of Saint ORLAN" in the 1990s. ORLAN'S facial map is captivating because
it is a conglomeration of features familiar to popular culture and Western
art history, yet made peculiar through surgical intervention.

While her performances are frequently mistaken for a form of beau-
tification, obsession with feminine perfection, or masochism, ORLAN
offers the following commentary on her art:

My work is not a stand against cosmetic surgery, but against the standards of beauty, against the dictates of a dominant ideology that impresses itself more and more on feminine (as well as masculine) flesh.

Cosmetic surgery is one of the areas in which man's power over woman can inscribe itself most strongly.

I would not have been able to obtain from the male surgeon what I obtained from my female surgeon; the former wanted, I think, to keep me "cute."[2]

ORLAN's remarks about the difficulty of finding surgeons willing to collaborate with her point to a key tension that I question and explore in this book – the contradiction between the transformative and imaginative *promises* of cosmetic surgery and the very real *limitations* to transformation imposed by both the cosmetic surgery industry and the body itself on those who seek out such surgeries. The ideology of cosmetic surgery promises patients and surgeons limitless opportunities to exercise individual agency within the surgical field, and yet the agency of both actors is constrained by the social, cultural, and biological limits imposed through the body's surface.

Using (cosmetic) surgical culture as its example, this book investigates the significance of surface to contemporary Western (and increasingly non-Western) cultures. The term "surgical culture"[3] was coined by Virginia Blum to describe the pervasive impact of cosmetic surgery on our conceptions of our bodies and identities; it provokes a seemingly inescapable surgical attitude toward those parts of our body that we do not like. Even though it can be invasive, painful, traumatic, and risky, and sometimes requires long periods of recovery, cosmetic surgery has become accepted as a reasonable option, if not an ideal solution, for addressing dissatisfactions with our bodies. Why is cosmetic surgery so easily assimilated within the Western cultural imaginary? How is such a physically traumatic surgical procedure – which commonly accomplishes changes that are visible only to the patient – domesticated and accepted?

• • •

To set about looking, to be seen, to make believe that one could be seen with successive images, straw images, of pseudos, right throughout my work is a curio of images of me, a myriad of photos, a flux, an explosion, a haemorrhage, a mass grave like the photo, a dysentery of images, like Adam born from mud, and filth like Lilith. (ORLAN, "The Future of the Body" conference)[4]

Skin is disappointing, in life all you have is your skin, there's a misdeal in human relationships because one is never what one has. I have an angel's skin, but I'm a jackal, a crocodile's skin, but I'm a little pooch, a black woman's skin, but I'm a white, a woman's skin, but I'm a man. I never have the skin of who I am, there's no exception to the rule because I am never what I have. (Eugénie Lemoine-Luccioni, cited by ORLAN, "The Future of the Body" conference)[5]

Photography and skin are the two primary surfaces of cosmetic surgery. The photograph is a promising surface, full of infinite transformative possibilities; the skin, on the contrary, is a less promising surface that, while capable of miraculous transformation, imposes limits on what surgery might accomplish. The fantasies projected onto these two surfaces facilitate an enthusiastic acceptance of cosmetic surgery globally in the twenty-first century. The excerpts from ORLAN's address to the "Future of the Body" conference at Science Gallery Dublin in June 2014, quoted above, offer a commentary on photography and skin that resonates with that of this book.

In a synthesis of themes that thread throughout her work, ORLAN identifies (mis)communication and (mis)recognition as central to her oeuvre. Perceptively linking together the body ("haemorrhage," "dysentery," birth, death) and the photograph in the first excerpt, ORLAN marks the photographic surface as a site of boundless and proliferating "flux." Yet this vast collection of images is only "make believe," an assortment of "pseudos" that ends up in a "mass grave" of representation. The endless misrecognition to which ORLAN here alludes is the result of an idealized disembodiment in the photographic image: we are compelled to create "make believe" images of ourselves because to refuse to do so would be even worse since, according to ORLAN, we would then be invisible.[6] The surface of the skin, idealized through the photographic surface, offers no consolation for this impasse since it too is deceptive.

In the second excerpt, ORLAN reads a passage from Lacanian psychoanalyst Eugénie Lemoine-Luccioni's *La robe: essaie psychanalytique sur le vêtement*, a passage that she read at the beginning of all her cosmetic surgical performances in the 1990s. Unlike the photograph, the skin is always already a "disappointment" because it exists as a limit, one that cannot accurately project an individual's interiority to the exterior world of others. The question of the skin is an ontological question, according to Lemoine-Luccioni and ORLAN's surgical oeuvre, because the skin one possesses will never be the subject one is. The skin is paradoxically both the entirety of our being ("in life all you have is your skin") and a deceptive mis-representational surface, a distortion of who we really are. In conjunction with the use and analysis of photography in ORLAN's lifetime of work, this passage frames ORLAN's cosmetic surgical performances of the early 1990s as a salient critique of the demand to interminably self-fashion our bodies as future photographs, a demand that is undermined by the skin as resistance, the skin as limit.

As an ordinary practice, cosmetic surgery grapples with the dissonance between the idealized photograph and the de-idealized skin that ORLAN exposes through her extraordinary work. ORLAN explains that she has no interest in particular materials or technologies, ancient or modern: she begins with a concept and then seeks to elucidate it through whatever means are most appropriate for the concept in the present.[7] She comments that her work in its entirety questions "the status of the body in society via cultural and socio-religious and political pressures ... in [her] flesh and blood."[8] She has chosen cosmetic surgery as the most appropriate means in the present because, as she explains, it is "very important to use cosmetic surgery to re-challenge, and to deregulate its codes and customs and its aesthetics, but also to de-dramatize it."[9] ORLAN challenges the practice of dramatically depicting the before and after of surgery through photographing the skin's surface and reveals the spaces in between these temporal moments.[10] According to Rachel Armstrong, a medical adviser and friend to ORLAN in the 1990s, she also exposes a "perverse picture of a future operating theatre."[11] The privatization of health care promises efficient and individually tailored options to its customers as active agents determining their own care, and cosmetic surgery is one example of such a system. Armstrong argues that ORLAN's spectacle demonstrates that such a model is not "utopian," but rather "peculiar, idiosyncratic, and psychotic"[12] because it is framed within neoliberal and individualist narratives supported by the ideology of cosmetic surgery, narratives that emphasize action and agency divorced from any ethical, political, or cultural contexts or engagements.

My inquiry is concerned with the cultural and individual fantasies buttressing these narratives of action and agency. A central component of this analysis is narrative interviews with seven women who have undergone cosmetic surgery at various ages (ranging from twenty-one to sixty-seven) and over different periods of time before our interview (ranging from three months to twenty-one years). These narratives elucidate the psychical and emotional effects of cosmetic surgery because they resist and complicate a commonplace interpretation of cosmetic surgery as a decision made exclusively to conform to mainstream beauty norms. Instead, like the extraordinary performances of ORLAN, these ordinary narratives offer rich commentary and critique of contemporary demands on embodiment, particularly the demand to construct ourselves as image through surface representations and transformations. Tigerlily had a partial face, neck, and eye lift at age sixty-seven. Melinda received a breast augmentation at age twenty-seven. Leah and Tonya underwent breast reduction and lift surgeries, at ages twenty-four and twenty-one, respectively. Diana had liposuction on her back and abdomen when she was thirty-five. Nicanor had a full face and eye lift at age forty-six. And finally, Victoria had been receiving ongoing chemical peels and laser treatments for acne beginning at age twenty-four. Five of the women identified as ethnically white (Tigerlily, Leah, Tonya, Diana, and Melinda), one identified as Hispanic-American (Nicanor), and one identified as Jewish (Victoria).[13] I introduce each of the interviewees in a bridging section between this preface and chapter 1, and specific details about their narratives follow in chapters 3 and 4, "The Photograph as Reminder, Evidence, and Promise" and "The Feminine Skin as Anxious Archipelago," which analyse their narratives through the concept of *surface imagination*.

Within the interviewees' stories, as well as in multiple narrative sites of cosmetic surgery from art to medicine to popular culture, the psychical effects of a body metamorphosis are presented as so powerful that the patient's *interior life* is transformed, with the promise of a better life and alleviation of psychic suffering.[14] Individual decisions to undergo cosmetic surgery are often made on the grounds that the surgery will be a means to overcome psychical distress, which contrasts with the notion that these decisions are an attempt to conform to a cultural ideal of beauty. The social and psychical circumstances in which the patient seeks out cosmetic surgery, and within which the practice flourishes culturally, are shaped by what I term *surface imagination*. This central concept is developed specifically through a psychoanalytic theoretical and methodological framework. *Surface imagination* refers to the fantasy that changes to our external appearance can transform our emotional and social lives. I explain this concept more fully in chapter 1 and develop it as an analytical tool throughout the book. The implications and complications of surface imagination fantasies are profound and widespread in contemporary Western cultures.

In the first chapter, I introduce the concept of *surface imagination* through establishing the theoretical and methodological frameworks for the book. The concept of surface imagination is used to examine cosmetic surgery's inescapable presence in North American culture. By thinking through individual surface imagination narratives of cosmetic surgery, it becomes possible to comment on larger social themes dealing with the significance of surface to fashioning identity and psyche. Beginning with an examination and questioning of the meaning and importance of surfaces to contemporary culture, I introduce cosmetic surgery as a key example of a cultural phenomenon produced by surface imagination fantasies. Thinking of cosmetic surgery as a surface imagination phenomenon moves analysis beyond the social/individual binary, as it considers these to be warp and weft of the primary surfaces of cosmetic surgery – the skin and the photograph. Thus, on the one hand, I argue against an analysis that focuses on the social at the expense of the individual, affective experience of cosmetic surgery; and on the other, an analysis that over-privileges the individual context and is not attentive enough to the power of surface imagination discourse produced by the cosmetic surgery industry. I establish that the conflation of the individual and the cultural contexts of cosmetic surgery happens because cosmetic surgery is a practice that is aligned with the quest for femininity and beauty. As such, the pursuit of cosmetic surgery is easily written off according to a rational, masculinist perspective that is embraced by feminists and non-feminists alike. The introductory chapter also articulates a method for reading interviews that is psychoanalytically informed, and that accounts for silences, leaps in logic, and parts of the interview that seem to be out of place within the context of my interview questions and our interview discussions. This psychoanalytic method for reading interview narratives enables me to better account for my position as interviewer and researcher and necessitates new practices for writing about narratives offered in the research interview setting, such as poetic transcription.

The second chapter, "From the Quest for Recognition to Surface Imagination Surgery," offers a genealogy of cosmetic surgery practice in the West. I link together the historical foundations of cosmetic surgery, psychoanalysis, and photography through their shared fragmented understanding of subjectivity, one that produced surface imaginations to comprehend and manage this fragmentation. Building on Sander Gilman's argument that psychoanalysis and cosmetic surgery hold inverse notions of cure, I discuss how psychoanalysis offers a cure for bodily symptoms through psychical work, while cosmetic surgery promises a cure for psychical problems through surgical work. Understanding the body as being in pieces and the skin as manipulable is necessary if the makeover is to enact its fantasies of transformation, and this chapter also offers an analysis of the makeover that connects its promises to the promises of cosmetic surgery and psychoanalysis. Finally, I introduce the topography of the photograph in cosmetic surgery through an examination of the transience of the photograph, the loss inaugurated by photography, and the before and after photograph in medical photography.

The third chapter, "The Photograph as Reminder, Evidence, and Promise," begins my interview analyses through theorizing the photograph as the idealized surface of cosmetic surgery. Photography was not a topic of interest in my initial research on cosmetic surgery, and yet I was intrigued that the interviewees told their stories in a highly visual manner that incorporated discussion of actual photographs and a way of seeing that is photographic. Unlike the mirror reflection, the photograph is an object that exists for others and enables cosmetic surgery patients to take themselves as other. As I elaborate in the following chapter, the old or manipulated photograph can be thought of as an idealized skin (or as portraying

an idealized skin) in its transformation of the three-dimensional flesh into
a two-dimensional image. Two inter-implicated sections in this chapter
discuss how photography structures surface imagination fantasies about
the body and examine how the interviewees used visual language and discussed photographs as a central component of their cosmetic surgery narratives. The first section examines how the interviewees talked about their
bodies photographically or in language borrowed from the study of art
and aesthetics. This discourse is borrowed from cosmetic surgeons,
whether it originates from what I call the surgeon-artist or the surgeon-
scientist.[15] It objectifies and fragments the body into many manipulable
pieces that can be altered or ameliorated, facilitating a necessary distance
from the experience of inhabiting a body that feels emotional and physical pain. This distance is crucial in mobilizing surface imagination fantasies that enable patients to imagine undergoing surgery in order to
correct visual flaws in their body. The second section of this chapter examines narratives about actual photographs, both the family snapshot
and glossy magazine layouts. These actual photographs contribute to the
patient's sense of possessing an embodied history and offer evidence that
their body looked different prior to surgery. For some interviewees, this
embodied past was something they wished to return to; for others, it was
a past they wished to surpass and change or at the very least document
as past. Magazine photographs provided a source of inspiration, both in
terms of how a body is supposed to look but also how the body will look
before and after cosmetic surgery. This chapter draws on Kaja Silverman's
critique of the ascendancy of vision in contemporary culture, and particularly on her discussion of the dangers and necessity of image idealization. Silverman's work helps me think about the interior and exterior of
the body in cosmetic surgery and how cosmetic surgery might be thought
of as an imperfect solution to psychical problems with one's body. I conclude this chapter with a return to the French performance artist ORLAN,
analysing the before and after photograph as it is ruptured by her surgical
performances, and incorporating Parveen Adams's insight that ORLAN's
work exposes the feminine body as an empty image.

The fourth chapter, "The Feminine Skin as Anxious Archipelago," examines the role of skin as the de-idealized surface of cosmetic surgery in the
interview narratives. I argue that the restorative and inscriptive capacities

of skin sustain the central surface imaginations of cosmetic surgery, and
that it is seductive to think of the skin's surface as infinitely alterable and customizable according to our wishes in a surface imagination culture. In
order to provide context for three auxiliary themes within the general
theme of skin in cosmetic surgery, I begin the chapter with a discussion
of the bodily ego and the unconscious in Freudian psychoanalysis, relating it to Didier Anzieu's extension of this theory into his metaphor of the
skin ego. The skin ego is a metaphor that considers the psychical functions
of the skin as barrier, container, and interface, and the relation between
the biological and the cultural. The first theme I identify in the discussions of skin is that our first experiences of contingency and accident are
through our skins. Thus, cosmetic surgery can be a way of negotiating
this contingency, and yet it also challenges the patient because the results
of surgery are unpredictable. Through this theme, I explore the accidental and mysterious skin-happenings in the interview narratives. The second theme examines the skin as the location where the interior and
exterior worlds meet. This is the realm in which the patient most frequently justifies her decision to have surgery in psychological terms, by
explaining that her interior perception of what she looks like does not
match with how she appears to the world. The final theme of this chapter analyses the relation between skin and time. The skin may be suddenly
marked by time, which is the experience of the cut or scar, or it may be
gradually marked by time, which is the experience of the wrinkle or sag.
Before concluding this chapter, I include a speculative digression on the
possible implications of surface imagination as a concept for an analysis
of sex reassignment surgeries. This speculation branches out from Jay
Prosser's work on transsexual autobiographies and second skins, as well
as Nikki Sullivan's exploration of the "wrong body" narrative – a narrative often shared by cosmetic surgery patients and used in mainstream discourses to explain transsexuality. By way of conclusion, I present Renata
Salecl's analysis that the deliberate cut in the skin can be thought of as a
response to the absence of the big Other. This cut attempts to fix the subject in time by establishing the skin as one's own.

The final chapter connects the concept of surface imagination to other
ways of understanding body transformations and psychical life in contemporary culture. When cosmetic surgery is an option for addressing

one's complaints about one's body, the way that all bodies are understood is fundamentally altered. Bodies come to be seen as a key component of one's social and cultural capital, and the way that we think about bodily improvement is structured by capitalist demands to market one's self to others. In this concluding chapter, I consider why surface imagination fantasies are so seductive, and what consequences this has not only for those who undergo cosmetic surgery, but also for *all* of us living in a surface imagination culture.

SURFACE IMAGINATIONS

MAKING
INTRODUCTIONS

Grandmother and Mother (Nicanor, face and eye lift)

My grandmother on my mother's side
had lots of wrinkles.
And I detested her.
I never liked her – I never loved her.

I remember being very little
Telling my friends,
"The day I have as many wrinkles as my grandmother –
I will commit suicide."

Then my mother was the most vain person I have ever met in my life.

I sent her a letter (that was time of the letters)
I said I was planning to have this cosmetic surgery,
And she phoned me, and said: "I'll give you the $3000."
She never congratulated me because I had a PhD in engineering.

And, I did not love my mother.
There was always some criticism of how I looked, I couldn't win.

She tortured my life; I was unfortunately the only girl.
And, this continued, all my life.

All.
My.
Life.

I mean, she was so vain.

It took me more than the surgery probably to get over that.

I interviewed Tigerlily in her posh, downtown condo. This was the first interview I conducted, and I was nervous, not only because I wasn't sure whether my questions would solicit the information I was looking for but also because I was uncomfortable in the upscale location. Tigerlily's face, neck, and eye lift surgeries had occurred ten years before we met. She described this time as emotionally contradictory. While she was happy in a new relationship, she was unhappy with her appearance. Her decision to have cosmetic surgery came slowly, and she mulled over the options for roughly seventeen years before she entered a cosmetic surgeon's office. Clearly, something in my call for interviewees drew Tigerlily in, but her interview was set apart from the others by her repeated statements that there might not be much good material for my research in her story because she expected that most other women who underwent cosmetic surgery procedures would have significantly more "drama" attached to their stories than she did. Her interview emphasized being realistic about surgical outcomes as well as societal expectations about aging; she felt that this realism separated her from other women who had sought cosmetic surgery. Tigerlily said that while the aging process was strange, it was also normal and natural. At the same time, she considered cosmetic surgery to be an ordinary occurrence in the lives of the women around her, even though it was not a topic of extensive discussion among these women. Throughout her interview, she highlighted the elite status of cosmetic surgery. Tigerlily mentioned a friend's cosmetic surgery holiday to South Africa for procedures similar to hers, plus a safari, and highlighted the superiority of her surgeon, citing as evidence not only his skill but also his pretty and thin wife. She noted her willingness to travel to his clinic, even though there were very good options in her own city, and her ability to afford the luxury of staying overnight at the clinic after her surgery, rather than travelling back to her hotel room, as proof of her belonging to and engagement with this elite world. This tension between the ordinariness of cosmetic surgery and its exclusivity is one that Tigerlily held throughout the interview.

I felt more comfortable and relaxed during Melinda's interview than during Tigerlily's. We met in Melinda's home, located in an urban residential neighbourhood, and there were several breaks and pauses in the interview because Melinda's child was home and in and out of the living room as she had a bath, got a snack, and read to herself. The pauses gave me more time to reflect on the process of the interview and seemed to give Melinda space to expand on what she had said about her breast augmentation surgery before the breaks. She received breast implants three or four years before we met (she couldn't remember exactly when), when she was twenty-six or twenty-seven years old, and described her surgery as "very much" connected to her gender and sexuality. Like Tigerlily, Melinda distanced herself from other women who have cosmetic surgery, for two reasons: first, she envisioned that many women who have surgery do so because they have been convinced by socially imposed beauty norms and ideals; and second, she described her motivations for having surgery as originating from psychological trauma and her surgery itself as causing higher than average physical trauma. Her decision to have surgery was framed as the result of the end of an abusive relationship and of a wish to regain the larger breast size she had had when she was pregnant and breastfeeding her daughter. Having breast augmentation surgery was a way of taking control of her life and caring for herself, and she described her decisions as the "best ones," especially in terms of choosing a surgeon and type of implant. Complications after her surgery from anaesthesia and pain medication required Melinda to be hospitalized, and she described these outcomes as traumatic. She also became disillusioned with the surgeon. While she was very pleased with the results of her surgery, she expressed feeling politically conflicted about it, in terms of her identities as a mother, a leftist organizer, and a feminist, and even described feeling embarrassment and shame regarding her decision.

Leah underwent breast reduction surgery just over one year before we met. She had been considering this surgery for eight years before she sought out a surgical consultation. The paradox in Leah's interview is that she discussed her breast size as very inconvenient and uncomfortable (specifically in terms of buying clothing and body image), but her primary concern was the stretch mark scarring on her breasts (the result of rapid breast development in adolescence). This is paradoxical because the scars left behind after breast reduction surgery are usually significantly larger and more visible than stretch marks. Leah made her decision within a community of women, including her friends, her mother, and her boyfriend's mother, and received encouragement and emotional support for her decision from this community. Her surgeon, in contrast, she described as a "mechanic," who was "nice" but emotionally absent from the consultation appointments and treated Leah as an object to be manipulated. Leah idealized her mother's body – it was "cute" and "perfect" – and saw her mother as unable to sympathize with the feelings Leah experienced as a result of her breast size. Yet Leah explained that her mother's approval was necessary for her to feel confident about her decision to undergo breast reduction surgery, and, once obtained, this approval resulted in a brisk chain of events that led to her surgery. In contrast, Leah derived emotional support from her boyfriend's mother. She is very satisfied with her decision, and described her post-surgical breasts as less of a "burden" because they don't attract attention and she can shop for clothing easily. Leah described herself as not being "attached to" her breasts and employed particularly vivid visual metaphors and language to talk about her skin, which is more of a focal point in the interview than her breasts.

Like Leah, Tonya had breast reduction and lift surgery that was paid for by provincial health insurance. Her surgery took place nine years prior to our interview. However, unlike Leah, Tonya had not considered undergoing a breast surgery until she went to an appointment with a specialist (for a lump in her breast), who asked if she had ever thought about a breast reduction. This question initiated a series of consultation appointments. Tonya made significant efforts to contextualize her narrative within a broader social framework; so, for example, she was critical of the absence of a waiting period for a surgery that will make women's breasts fit into a cultural ideal, while other surgeries have long waiting lists (the example she offered was kidney transplant surgery). She found the experience of meeting with her surgeon in a consultation room objectifying and degrading, partly because of his distanced demeanour and partly because she had never shown her bare breasts to someone with the lights on. A pattern that emerged in Tonya's narrative was her lack of knowledge throughout the process. It is difficult to distinguish whether she was emphasizing the patronizing attitude of the surgeon, who disclosed information only if asked, or demonstrating her difference from other women who research cosmetic surgery and think about their decisions extensively and thoroughly. Tonya talked about her breasts in an exceptionally objectifying and distancing manner, describing her breasts as not a part of her, and taking delight in details of the surgery such as the removal of her nipple and its placement in a petri dish. Like Melinda, she expressed conflict between her identity as a feminist and her decision to undergo breast reduction surgery. Tonya noted the seemingly miraculous capability of the skin to heal and recover from traumatic experiences like cosmetic surgery. She felt ready to have surgery because she could clearly recall her recovery from a car accident that caused significant superficial trauma to her face and body. She was well cared for by her mother after her surgery, and very satisfied with the results, especially the low level of scarring. Tonya was able to express her sexuality more freely because her breast reduction surgery gave her a new ownership of her body. She described her post-surgical breasts as not belonging to her, so she marked them as her own through tattooing and piercing.

Most of the interviewees expressed an acceptance of their surgeries and decisions to have surgery, even if they were critical of their own motivations, social and cultural ideals for women's bodies, their surgeons, or some of their post-operative results (such as side effects). Diana's narrative stands out because she remained incisively critical of her decision to undergo liposuction on her abdomen and flanks, specifically because she was recovering from an eating disorder and felt that her decision to have surgery was not "mature" or "healthy." She had had liposuction three months before we met, and she was the only interviewee whose cosmetic surgeon was a woman. The liposuction process itself did not make Diana anxious, although she was afraid of being under general anaesthetic. More than any other interviewee, Diana discussed her surgery in a way that seemed disembodied and highly intellectualized; in her attempts to rationalize her decision, she equivocated and judged her actions harshly. Her narrative was marked not only by this striking ambivalence, but also by her use of the concept "body image." She explained her experience of being diagnosed with an eating disorder extensively to me as though I would not be familiar with the diagnosis, and noted that she was relatively far along in the recovery process. Because I didn't comment on or respond to her judgment of her liposuction as unhealthy or immature, it seemed that Diana made an effort to explain to me how her surgery gave solid evidence that she wasn't recovered enough and that she did not view her body in a realistic manner (so to Diana, her body image was inaccurate). From Diana's perspective, her decision to undergo liposuction, while partially successful in alleviating her insecurities about her body, was a last resort option that was inappropriate for a person in recovery. Diana gave a particularly arresting narrative of the period of time after her surgery: she described being liberated from having a body image because she couldn't visualize her body in her mind anymore. This interview was difficult ecause Diana's story raised many questions for me about the ethics of cosmetic surgery (and her surgeon in particular). Diana told her story in a way that emphasized that she underwent liposuction even though she did not think it was healthy for her as a person recovering from an eating disorder. While it was unclear whether Diana told her surgeon that she was in recovery, this interview challenged the claims of the cosmetic surgery industry that they carry out a careful and thorough psychological screening of patients to ensure that patients do not undergo surgery for what Diana characterized as the "wrong" reasons.

Nicanor, who was introduced at the beginning of this section through a poetic transcription, was interviewed under the least ideal conditions for me as an interviewer. On the day that I interviewed her, I had lost my voice and forgotten my interview questions; however, and perhaps because of these less than ideal circumstances, this was the most compelling and smoothest interview that I conducted for this project. Nicanor had a face and eye lift twenty years before I interviewed her, when she was forty-six years old. She had immigrated to Canada from South America, and then found herself as a professional in a workplace that was male dominated (she and the secretary were the only women in a company of about five hundred employees), sexist, and ageist. Her decision to have cosmetic surgery was a response to this workplace. Because she was over-qualified for her position and the men above her were "incompetent" and unqualified, she wanted to advance in her career and felt that looking younger would increase her opportunities. While she found the recovery period very unpleasant – she could not read and took a long time to recover from the effects of local anaesthesia and sedatives – she thought her surgeon was very professional and gentlemanly and was satisfied with the results (although she hastened to add that she would never undergo another cosmetic surgery procedure because of the recovery period). This narrative was compelling, for two reasons. First, Nicanor emphasized repeatedly that her decision to get cosmetic surgery was completely out of character for her and that it shocked her family and close friends. She even told me that she thought I should have asked her to tell me more about why it was so out of character. She gave as an example that she didn't think it was politically compatible to refuse to buy flowers because they are grown in places like Venezuela, where people don't have enough to eat, *and* accept cosmetic surgery as a viable option. I found this statement interesting because it made me realize that each of the women I had interviewed to this point (Tigerlily, Leah, Melinda, Tonya, and Diana) had described their decisions as uncharacteristic in some way or another, so I had not noticed this as a unique feature of Nicanor's interview in the same way that she did. Second, Nicanor's narrative of her surgeries was situated in a broader narrative of embodiment that existed as a matrilineal pattern from her grandmother to her mother to Nicanor. The only information Nicanor gave about her grandmother, as described in the poetic transcription above, was that she was "detested" and wrinkled. In contrast, Nicanor offered a great deal of evidence of her mother's superficiality and vanity, her unfair and lifelong criticisms of her only daughter for not meeting her ideals of femininity (thinness, delicacy, prettiness, fairness), and her wholehearted support of her decision to get a facelift, which stood in marked contrast to her indifference about Nicanor's attaining a doctoral degree.

Victoria is the only interviewee who underwent procedures that fall within the fastest growing segment of the cosmetic surgery market: quick, relatively inexpensive, and non-invasive treatments for the skin's surface that involve chemicals, lasers, and injectables.[1] She had struggled with acne for years before she began to be treated with a chemical peel once a month and received laser treatments on problem areas as needed. She began these procedures at age twenty-five, approximately one year before our interview and after she ended an unsatisfying romantic relationship. She planned on receiving these treatments for the next five years, which she hoped would be a long-term solution for her acne. Victoria described her treatments as the penultimate resort before seeking out Accutane (isotretinoin), a medication with many side effects and risks (particularly for birth defects) that requires patients capable of becoming pregnant to take birth control medication concurrently (something Victoria did not want to do). The chemical peels and laser treatments fit within a carefully constructed and maintained regime of activities that Victoria followed in order to keep her acne to a minimum. The regime also included exercise, severe diet restrictions, adequate sleep, stress reduction, and several skin care rules (for example, not sleeping with makeup on). Victoria emphasized that she was committed to taking care of herself and that these treatments were a substantial part of this commitment, in terms of both time and expense. However, her expressed self-commitment conflicted with her desires to eat foods like burgers, french fries, and chocolate milkshakes and take a more relaxed approach to caring for her skin, as well as her mother's constant surveillance and policing of Victoria's eating and skin care habits. Victoria emphasized that her mother was extremely vigilant and concerned about her skin, and because they lived together this had an impact on her everyday life. In addition to Victoria's involvement in a significant and under-researched area of cosmetic surgery, this interview stood out because of how she situated her treatments as necessary to achieve ideals of heterosexual femininity. Perhaps as a result, she described her female friends as jealous competitors who were not compassionate about her rigorous commitment to maintaining her body and face, and her mother as a policing figure who was particularly concerned about the effects of Victoria's skin on finding a male partner.

SURFACE IMAGINATIONS

1

Cosmetic surgery is too complex a cultural phenomenon to be studied from the social or the psychical perspective alone. This book examines the two simultaneously, even while recognizing that these dimensions are often inchoate and in conflict with one another. This approach involves, on the one hand, holding together the complexities and uniqueness of individual cosmetic surgery experiences and respecting those who undergo and practise cosmetic surgery, and, on the other, formulating a rigorous critique of cosmetic surgery as an industry. I do not see those who have cosmetic surgery as naive victims, but neither do I see them as exercising unfettered agency in their decisions. Likewise, surgeons are neither benevolent miracle workers committed to a philanthropic project nor are they the despotic men of Ira Levin's *The Stepford Wives*, manipulating women into their fantasies; instead, surgeons navigate a complex ideological and historical terrain, although they are not the focus of this book.

Through a decade of following cosmetic surgery in popular culture and having conversations with patients and others interested in cosmetic surgery, I have learned that while cosmetic surgery carries many psychical and social benefits, any engagement with the profession is far from utopic. This is the case for surgeons, but it is especially so for patients. Although most of the women I interviewed became comfortable in their own skins through cosmetic surgery, they were confronted with imperfect options that were the result of photographically dominated mandates and ideals pursued by the cosmetic surgery profession. They negotiated a profession that places all participants in rigidly gendered roles with few options for surgical outcomes, as well as a cultural context that trivializes and devalues femininity and the pursuit of beauty. As a consequence, even though the interviewees overall were very satisfied with the results of their surgeries, these results were not perfect and their stories are not uniformly positive. The complaints present in their narratives, and denoted by scars, numbness, and flaws in surgical outcomes, register as necessary failures to obtain a desired result.

Nonetheless, most of the women believed their lives had improved as a result of their procedures and therefore regarded these complications as a worthwhile compromise for attaining a social and psychical objective through surgery. They found greater enjoyment in their romantic, familial, and friend relationships, they were more successful at work, and their experience of inhabiting their bodies in this world was easier after their surgeries. This is consistent with large-scale psychological studies of cosmetic surgery conducted both within and outside the industry, which indicate that what might be considered a small cosmetic change can have significant effects on the lives of patients.[1] These large-scale studies and the narratives in this book offer inklings into the contradictory conditions and outcomes of cosmetic surgery in contemporary North America.

This chapter is concerned with these contradictions, using them to better situate surface imagination fantasies within cosmetic surgery. In order to differentiate my analysis from prior work, I begin with a discussion of the diverse field of feminist cosmetic surgery studies. I then move into a more comprehensive discussion of the book's central concept, *surface imagination*, elaborating on the insights that can be gleaned from psychoanalysis to flesh out the concept of surface imaginations, before moving on to explain the methodological innovations necessary to interpret the narratives of cosmetic surgery.

Feminist Cosmetic Surgery Studies

Feminist cosmetic surgery studies is a vibrant, complex, and interdisciplinary field.[2] Here I outline some important strands of debate within the field to situate and distinguish my work, since my approach draws on literatures and methodologies that differ from the majority of feminist works on cosmetic surgery.

Feminist researchers have understood cosmetic surgery as a "dilemma," according to Kathy Davis, and many feminist analyses of the practice attempt a "feminist balancing act."[3] The industry and practice of cosmetic surgery is ripe for feminist critique as sexist, racist, ageist, and fatphobic, and has been roundly censured on these grounds. Yet such critical approaches, which tend to focus on the cosmetic surgery industry rather than on the individuals who undergo surgery, risk labelling all recipients of cosmetic surgery as naive victims of false consciousness and patriarchal culture. Take, for example, this excerpt from Susan Bordo's "Material Girl: The Effacements of Postmodern Culture": "The rhetoric of choice and self-determination and the breezy analogies comparing cosmetic surgery to fashion accessorizing are deeply mystifying. They efface not only the inequalities of privilege, money, and time that prohibit most people from indulging in these practices, but also the desperation that characterizes the lives of those who do."[4] This is an important critique of the ways in which the contemporary cosmetic surgery industry characterizes its work (as parallel to the work of fashion[5]), yet Bordo's characterization of those who seek out cosmetic surgery as "indulgent" and "desperate" undermines the critique through its latent misogyny.[6] What these analyses accomplish is a discerning critique of the oppressive underpinnings of cosmetic surgery's proliferation; what they do less well is account for the ways in which individual women experience positive change in their lives through engaging with cosmetic surgery as a body practice.

On the other hand, the use of patient narratives of cosmetic surgery as evidence of patients' agency and ability to negotiate with the system has not been wholly convincing either. In particular, there is a danger of overestimating the degree of autonomy patients possess when engaging with an industry that is thoroughly shaped by white supremacist-capitalist-patriarchy, to use bell hooks's apt phrasing. Kathy Davis's *Reshaping the Female Body: The Dilemma of Cosmetic Surgery* (1995) is emblematic of this approach.[7] Here, she recalls the irritated and dismissive response to her work that she received at a feminist conference, which was in sharp contrast to the positive response that philosopher Kathryn Pauly Morgan received for her paper, which characterized cosmetic surgery recipients as "Stepford Wives" and the practice as a technological colonization of

women's bodies.[8] According to Davis, presenting women who had undergone cosmetic surgery as active agents taking control of their lives was
unthinkable and unacceptable within feminist scholarly communities of the
early 1990s. While Davis's work is sometimes critiqued as overly trusting
of the patients' accounts, privileging action and rational choice, and too
optimistic about the effects of cosmetic surgery,[9] her approach was ground-
breaking in its time. It was the result of qualitative interview research (previous feminist writing about cosmetic surgery was not) and resisted the
latent (and easy) misogyny of analyses that positioned women as "cultural
dopes" (in Davis's phrasing).[10] The majority of feminist analyses of cosmetic surgery attempt to strike a balance between criticizing and listening
to women who have undergone cosmetic surgery, but the more entrenched
positions described above reveal the dilemma of cosmetic surgery for feminist scholars.

The 2000s marked a departure from the question "Why do women
undergo cosmetic surgery?" toward conceiving of cosmetic surgery as a
"culture" of its own, symptomatic of contemporary Western cultures,
especially in terms of consumerism and globalization. Rebecca Huss-
Ashmore, a medical anthropologist, argues that Western deference to
medical expertise and scientific explanations makes cosmetic surgery an
ideal "ritual setting." Huss-Ashmore holds that women engage in the
practice because it provides a "culturally meaningful" space for self-
transformation and locating an authentic self.[11] Virginia Blum writes of
a "culture of cosmetic surgery" or a "surgical culture" that fuels narcissistic pursuits and the overvaluation of the body through offering surgery
as a response to the demand for attractiveness, while paradoxically
dematerializing the body through refusing its vulnerability.[12] Cressida
Heyes holds that cosmetic surgery is a method of self-transformation that
is shaped by a conception of the body as failed within a culture of normalization, but that the individual can be vindicated through active work
on the body to reveal the truth of the inner self.[13] Meredith Jones situates
cosmetic surgery within a broader "makeover culture" that values the
process of becoming over the state of being and encourages individuals to
engage in ongoing and visible work on the self.[14] These approaches, which
situate cosmetic surgery as a culture or as operating within cultural frameworks, offer valuable and necessary nuance to understandings of the prac-

tice. They avoid becoming enmeshed within a debate about whether cosmetic surgery is "good" or "bad" for women and, instead, attempt to grasp what cultural factors make cosmetic surgery a viable option for so many women (and increasingly, men).

In more recent works, Debra Gimlin and Bernadette Wegenstein attempt to bridge questions about why women undergo cosmetic surgery with cultural analyses of the practice. Gimlin's *Cosmetic Surgery Narratives: A Cross-Cultural Analysis of Women's Accounts* (2012) offers a comparative analysis of women's experiences of cosmetic surgery in the United States and Britain, arguing that the strategies that American and British women use to justify undergoing a cosmetic surgery are shaped by their differing national health care systems in conjunction with local and global cultural values.[15] She demonstrates that where American women's narratives tend to be shaped by a consumer approach to health care,[16] British women's narratives are shaped by an understanding of healthcare as a means to level social differences and rely on local understandings of cosmetic surgery as an "entitlement" that is earned through moral living (being a "good" person or "suffering" from the body).[17] Gimlin's is one of just a few studies of cosmetic surgery that uses a cross-cultural approach.[18]

Wegenstein's book, *The Cosmetic Gaze*, proposes the idea of a cosmetic gaze that structures modes of looking at bodies informed by techniques and discourses of body modification.[19] The cosmetic gaze is obsessed with transformation of the body to match a fixed, true interior self, and imagines this transformation as possible only through practices of cutting by the scalpel or the cursor.[20] The "machinic suture" refers to the operation through which a true self is made visible through the "performative influence of augmented realities."[21] Wegenstein traces the history of the cosmetic gaze through practices such as physiognomy to demonstrate how the same gaze that was used to demonstrate racial superiority through composite photography is now being "repackaged by technology [e.g., cosmetic surgery] into a socially acceptable care of the self."[22] This incisive analysis of body modification helps explain why individuals might engage with an industry like cosmetic surgery, even as it diminishes their authority and agency. Wegenstein's work complements mine, although I understand these patterns of looking to be situated in modern visual practices, an evaluation that is informed by the work of such historians as Elizabeth Haiken and Sander Gilman, and theorists such as Anne Anlin Cheng.[23]

Surface Imagination Fantasies and Psychoanalytic Possibilities

My engagement with the field is inspired by similar questions, particularly about the seductive qualities of idealized representations of beauty and the psychical suffering that women frequently report as a key cause of seeking out cosmetic surgery. However, while my work in this book is informed by debates and discussions within feminist cosmetic surgery studies, it takes a markedly distinct approach in order to ask these questions differently. Feminist analyses, particularly those informed primarily by sociology, are haunted by a gap between the narratives of cosmetic surgery offered by recipients, surgeons, and popular culture, and the visceral corporeality of surgery itself. To be blunt, cosmetic surgery is a physically traumatic experience for the vulnerable human body. It can be difficult to understand why someone would submit to its invasive and violent force. Narratives of cosmetic surgery, including television programs inspired by "makeover culture," usually move silently past the technical and sometimes brutal details of these procedures. Although television shows like *Extreme Makeover* and *The Swan* contain segments that are filmed in the operating room and show some of the cosmetic surgery, these segments are carefully edited to reduce hours of surgery into a clip of two to three minutes. They do not linger over or zoom in on some of the most violent interventions of cosmetic surgery, such as forcing an implant underneath the chest wall or repeatedly ramming a metal tube into the body during liposuction.

When we compare the popularity of *Extreme Makeover* with the response to ORLAN's surgical performances, in which viewers watched her surgeries in galleries worldwide via live satellite, we see a stark contrast. Few original audience members remained until the end of ORLAN's forty-five-minute performance; they were simply too horrified and sickened to continue to watch as her body was cut open and operated upon.[24] In contrast, *Extreme Makeover* (2002–2007, four seasons) has inspired several other cosmetic surgery reality television series (*Plastic Surgery: Before and After,* 2002–2008, five seasons; *Dr 90120,* 2004–2008, six seasons; *The Swan,* 2004, two seasons; and *Miami Slice,* 2004, one season). Apparently, viewers cannot get enough of these televised transformations – it was even rumoured that the widely criticized reality show *The Swan* was planning a reunion show in 2014.

The most recognizable visual referent of cosmetic surgery is the photograph, especially the before and after images that depict the patient before her procedure and after she has recovered from it. The fixation on the before and after images, which are ubiquitous in cosmetic surgery culture, rather than the "in-between" space in which the procedures take place, is central to understanding contemporary cosmetic surgery, culturally and psychically. Shows like *Extreme Makeover* present the viewer not with an accurate representation of the work involved in cosmetic surgery but with simulacral images that diminish the corporeality of this work. As I discuss later, while my interviewees narrate their surgeries as a part of their embodied history, they do so not so much as a means of becoming but rather as a means of fixing the body into an idealized time and form.[25]

Consistent across many analyses of cosmetic surgery is an inability to bridge this gap between event and effect. This is because this gap is not a conscious one, but one that is structured by an unconscious logic. For this reason, psychoanalysis offers an incomparable approach to understanding this gap. It makes possible an ethical consideration of the relationship between the socio-cultural dimensions of life and the singularity of the individual's experience within that socio-cultural milieu. An explanation of the social and cultural factors that shape the existence of a proliferating phenomenon like cosmetic surgery is essential to any discussion of the practice; however, this explanation alone is unable to hold narratives of cosmetic surgery without crushing the parts that resist socio-cultural interpretation through their singularity. A socio-cultural explanation can address only part of the interviewees' narratives. This type of analysis is in danger of omitting or considering as aberrations the parts of those narratives that don't fit within a conscious logic and appear inconsistent and incoherent; since the narratives shared in this book are about singular experiences of embodiment, it is often the case that they are non-linear and don't make sense. These difficult parts of the narratives can be held more gently through a psychoanalytic approach.

This book holds that understanding the way in which fantasy sustains the practice of cosmetic surgery can bridge the gap between the event and the effect of cosmetic surgery, as well as between the socio-cultural and the individual. In psychoanalysis, the fantasy has been defined in two ways: first, as a conscious product of the imagination that represents a wish-fulfillment; and second, as a mental representation that is formed unconsciously through the subject's relation to their internal and external worlds.[26] The latter definition has often been distinguished as "phantasy," through the German "phantasie," although in North America the two meanings have merged into the same word: "fantasy." My analysis is primarily concerned with the latter definition of fantasy, which has been taken up in Lacanian psychoanalysis as the means through which we "learn how to desire."[27] Our fantasies are, paradoxically, a defence against the imagined desire of the Other. The Other exists within the dimension that Lacan called the Symbolic, which means it is a field structured by cultural ideologies and language; as such, the Other is structured around a lack that fantasy attempts to conceal. A psychoanalytic approach can address the unconscious processes that structure the cultural *and* individual narratives of cosmetic surgery. The psychoanalytic concept of fantasy also helps to collapse the binary between surface and depth that is implicit in those analyses of cosmetic surgery that situate the cultural milieu within which cosmetic surgery flourishes as superficial and catering to image ideals, and differentiate the superficial from the deeper issues of structural oppression and emotional distress.

What happens within this gap between event and effect, where a relatively undetectable alteration to the body effects a significant change in the life of the cosmetic surgery recipient? While the representations of cosmetic surgery in popular culture are increasingly focused on extreme transformations and multiple surgeries, in the case of most patients, their cosmetic surgical changes are difficult or even impossible for others to detect.[28] It is not the case that the majority of cosmetic surgery patients undergo a radical transformation in order to make themselves irresistibly attractive to others in their personal and professional lives. Rather, for the majority of people in her life, the cosmetic surgery patient remains the same in terms of her appearance. And yet most patients still report feeling that their lives have changed, often dramatically.[29] Cosmetic surgery is obtained by the individual and flourishes culturally in social and psychical circumstances that are shaped by what I term *surface imagination*.

Surface imagination is a concept that refers to the powerful fantasy that a change to the exterior can enhance or alter the interior; in other words, the exterior creates and takes precedence over the interior. It is the seduction of surface imagination fantasies that creates the conditions in which cosmetic surgery patients' lives improve while their appearance remains relatively the same. Surface imaginations structure social and psychical life in the consumer-driven West where the condition and appearance of the exterior is seen as an indicator of interior qualities and values. Connected to the biopolitical imperative to care for the individual, hermetic self, surface imagination fantasies offer inspiration to, and proof of, the subject's dramatic narrative of care and success in the project of self-creation. To say that in the current moment surfaces matter is not to make a moral judgment, and therefore the concept of surface imagination must be separated from the kinds of popular media analyses that critique contemporary Western societies as superficial or fake. The devaluing of a concerted and intentional interest in the body and its appearance has a long history in Western philosophy, which has privileged the mind and separated it from the body.[30] Surface imagination takes the body's surface seriously, as a medium that is neither interior nor exterior but continuous. Precisely because of that Möebian quality, the surface is a site of fantasy and projection. Joanna Frueh writes of the "soul-and-mind-inseparable-from-body,"[31] which has inspired me to theorize the surface not as shallow and trivial, but profound and vital – the very material out of which identities are fashioned.

Applied to cosmetic surgery, surface imagination shores up the fantasy that changing the surfaces of our bodies will change or improve our identities, and consequently, supports the possibility and promise of the cosmetic surgery industry that our bodies are infinitely transformable and controllable according to our desires. The mutable body promised and fantasized through the surface imagination of cosmetic surgery is first and foremost a controllable body.

Cosmetic surgery is a cultural effect of surface imagination, and we can learn more about how contemporary embodiment is broadly understood through individual experiences within the specific practice of cosmetic surgery. Particularly significant in current understandings of embodiment in North America is the persistent belief of advanced capitalism that psychical and social suffering can be alleviated through our body's surface, especially through self-fashioning or transforming it. Cosmetic surgery exists alongside other cultural products of surface imaginations, such as ego psychology, pornography, and home renovation. These exemplify how surface imagination logic influences the understanding of the psychological, sexual, and domestic realms of contemporary life. Ego psychology, which assumes a rational and fully conscious subject, envisions transformations of the self through a manipulation of the psyche's surface (the ego). If the subject can strengthen or re-route the ego's functioning, the subject's psychical life will become whole and unproblematic. The pornographic surface imagination creates sexual life as a repetition of sexual acts focused not on the touch-sensations of pleasure but on a stylized aesthetics of sex. Pleasure is visual, not tactile, in pornography, and thus the transformation of the body through pleasure occurs through the surface of the magazine, television, computer, or mobile phone. Home renovations, and the proliferation of popular media and cultural practices devoted to this activity, exist in a relationship with cosmetic surgery that is more obvious and parallel than pornography and ego psychology. Transforming one's domestic space, whether through major structural renovations or minor changes to decor, is correlated with positive emotional and psychological responses. These responses occur because the interior of the home has been aligned with the inhabitants' personalities and needs, which are projected out into the transformation of the home. Ego psychology, pornography, and home renovations are not the only cultural products of surface imaginations, but they are illustrative of the range and scope of surface imaginations in contemporary culture.

The question of the surface is important to understanding contemporary Western (and increasingly, non-Western) cultures. Anne Anlin Cheng argues that there is a profound ontological quality to the modern surface that is often overlooked or looked at with suspicion due to the devaluation of visuality within Western philosophy.[32] Cosmetic surgery is a cultural phenomenon where this ontological quality can be observed, especially through its primary surfaces of the photograph and the skin. The photograph represents an idealized surface for the cosmetic surgery industry since it can depict whatever the patient or surgeon might desire, without pain or contingency. The photograph is thus a magical object, capable of representing the past, present, and future of the patient's skin, which supports the fragmentation and objectification of the body necessary to imagine an aesthetic surgical intervention. In contrast, the skin is the textile surface upon which that surgical intervention occurs; but it is not as easily manipulated as the photograph. The skin is a de-idealized surface for the cosmetic surgery industry, because it is subject to the exigencies of time and healing. Both the photographic and dermal surfaces are sites where the socio-cultural realm of ideals and norms and the psychical realm of fantasy and seduction meet.

Within this milieu, skin is transformed from a house for the body's contents into a garment or window dressing that displays the self to the world.[33] Cosmetic surgery's central fantasy is that the body is mutable and can be altered at will to suit the current demands of the patient. Photography supports cosmetic surgery in sustaining this fantasy, which re-imagines skin as a garment or textile. In contemporary North America, cultures of surface have risen to primacy over cultures of depth, partially due to the invention and development of modern photography in the mid-nineteenth century. Skin is a marker of one's mental and physical health and a source of personal capital, and as a result, great attention is paid to the skin's appearance. In other words, skin is a surface that mediates and is mediated: we may write our own skins, but our skins are read by others, often with the appearance that there is nothing to us but skin. However, as a biological, social, and psychical surface, skin can never possess the perfection and capacity to transform of the photograph. This is a central disappointment and dilemma for the cosmetic surgery industry, and is experienced as such by patients and surgeons. Nevertheless, and perhaps because of this, the cosmetic surgery industry is burgeoning and an increasingly diverse population is interpellated into the surface imagination fantasies promised by cosmetic surgery.

The theoretical, methodological, and historical contexts within which I formulate the concept of surface imagination are varied and sometimes contradictory. This mirrors the strange and conflicting experience of privileging surface in contemporary culture. This privileging provides both a satisfaction and a rift because the surface doesn't seem to hold all that it promises in surface imagination fantasies. By focusing on the functions of photography and of skin in cosmetic surgery narratives, this book explores the surface imagination fantasy of the mutable body, which is premised on the belief that transforming the body alleviates psychic suffering – that there is an intimate relationship between the body's surface and the body's interior in which aspects of the interior are not only expressed on the surface, but the transformation of the surface can alter the interior. Such an understanding represents a devaluing of the interior as easily manipulable, as long as the correct surface techniques are deployed. The pre-eminence of the visual senses in contemporary Western cultures foregrounds the significance of surface to cosmetic surgery narratives, and to contemporary culture more broadly.

I use multiple methods from the social sciences and the humanities to explore these ideas. In considering the culture of cosmetic surgery, I combine interviewing and critical content analysis through an interdisciplinary methodology informed by psychoanalytic theory. These methods complement each other and seek to reveal each other's gaps. To accurately situate the narratives of cosmetic surgery that I include, it is important to begin with a detailed historical, ideological, and cultural analysis of cosmetic surgery in the West. Through content analysis of popular culture texts depicting ordinary women's decisions to have cosmetic surgery, and the historical and cultural context of cosmetic surgery, I am able to situate the practice as it is understood from both a general and specific vantage point. Content analysis of popular culture accounts contextualizes the interviews and guides a reading and rereading of these accounts of cosmetic surgery in light of the narratives that emerge in these interviews. It also facilitates an understanding of the cultural meaning behind cosmetic surgery and its relationship to skin and psyche.

I wish to interrogate the common assumption that interviewing is most appropriate for research in the social sciences and is ill-suited for research within the humanities and cultural studies. I am particularly interested in the ethics of combining interview methods with psychoanalytic methodologies as an academic, rather than as an analyst, because I am convinced that interviewing offers possibilities that are not present when a researcher studies only text. In her doctoral dissertation about the recovery movement, Erica Meiners concurs with my suspicions and concerns about focusing on text to the exclusion of such social science methods as interviewing when studying cultural phenomena like the recovery movement or cosmetic surgery. Meiners decided to include participant observation alongside textual analysis because she "became dissatisfied with [her] own ability to suture text: there was no friction."[34] Working with text alone makes it easier to distance oneself from the person who wrote it and to "suture" texts together in a way that is pleasing and comfortable for the researcher. Such suturing is more difficult when one is working with interviewees.

Psychoanalysis and Social Science
Interview Methodologies

The lyrebird is an Australian creature, almost a strange peacock with a steely grey body and tail feathers flanked on either side with an ostentatious whorl. In order to attract a mate, the lyrebird sings a tune that consists of every notable birdsong, forest noise, or human-generated sound the bird has ever heard, in a sequence composed by the bird. The lyrebird faithfully mimics these noises in timbre and resonance, and repeats them exactly as they were originally heard: the impersonation is so good that it fools practically all other creatures who have the privilege of eavesdropping on the vanishing bird's song.

The researcher who interviews is not a lyrebird.[35] She has neither the faculties to reproduce the talk of the interview accurately (memory, experience, the unconscious will intervene), nor the technology (even the best recording will fail us at least once, often when we need it the most). Trinh T. Minh-Ha writes that "for many of us the best way to be neutral is to copy reality meticulously,"[36] in other words, the model offered by the lyrebird. It is tempting to believe in the promises of positivism that interviewing is a way to hear the real voice of the interviewee, which may then be re-presented to others as a truthful depiction of what *really* happened in the interview and in the world, without the contamination of the researcher's bias. However, neither the interviewee nor the researcher is able to fully capture the experiences of the interviewee in language, nor can they express an absolute "truth" about the interviewee's story. I go beyond this positivist position in this book, and try to open up a different kind of space for the interviews in my research, one that is receptive to the partial truths, effects of retroactive reflection, and impossibilities of language that surface imagination culture tries to mask in favour of wholeness and impermeability.

– and I would have to affirm this uncertainty: is a translated interview a written or spoken object?

Interview: an antiquated device of documentary. Truth is selected, reviewed, disputed and speech is always tactical.[37]

What is the interview? The word likely comes from Old French, and means something like "to see one another."[38] But how does this become possible? "Interview" is a word that grasps hold of myriad experiences and encounters. It is at once an encounter and an exchange (a seeing of one another) that becomes a transcript, translated (an object). The interview, once transcribed, fixes a story into stillness of print, yet breathes life into the research as it is read. Interview narratives offer an enrichment of a project that is unavailable to the researcher without an encounter with another person. As researchers, we have an obligation to the interviewees through our co-construction of the interview-gift.

Using a psychoanalytically informed methodology to research surface imagination cultures through the relationships between cosmetic surgery, photography, and skin presents two major methodological issues. First, how can psychoanalysis be used to inform and complement postmodern qualitative methodologies, especially interviewing? What does this hybrid interview methodology look like? While an abundance of scholarship takes up psychoanalysis as a critical theoretical approach to studying culture, rarely does an author articulate the process or the effect of this approach itself in relation to the research. And second, how does a psychoanalytic methodology open up possible understandings of the interview and why does it compel the researcher to use innovative methods like poetic transcription to re-present the interviews?

In the collection *Framer/Framed*, Trinh interrogates the category of "scholarly" for academics, exposing it as a normative framework. She implies that the creation and boundary maintenance of this category limits what counts as "theory" through establishing norms about theoretical style and contents.[39] To extend her hyperbole, sanitized scholarship excises and disposes of the personal, affective, and sensual experiences of research, maintaining the boundaries of public/private, objective/subjective, as well as the distinctions between disciplines. Trinh goes so far as to say that although interdisciplinary work is presently chic, what counts as interdisciplinary research is frequently work that simply collects the disciplines together, side by side. This diminishes the radical threat that interdisciplinarity poses to academic scholarship and to the notions of expertise and ownership, which Trinh calls a "politics of pluralist exchange."[40] Disciplinary boundaries are sustained by methodological explanations and limitations as a defence against the anxiety generated by the often overwhelming experience of conducting research about other people and the difficulties in depicting another's story.

Psychoanalytic theory can enrich qualitative research methodologies, and in particular, interview methodologies. The research experience is often a conflicted emotional and psychical encounter between the researcher, their object(s) of study, and their theoretical and methodological frameworks. Sometimes scholars seek to minimize the affective dimension of research, choosing to understand it as an interference with research process. Occasionally (as in some feminist methodologies), the analysis of the subjective elements of research becomes a confessional list of identity qualifiers describing the researcher and the researched. Pierre Bourdieu holds that a researcher should "observe the effects produced on the observation, on the description of the thing observed, by the situation of the observer – to uncover all the pre-suppositions inherent in the *theoretical* posture."[41] This is an appealing aspiration, but it could also be manifested by a researcher as a defensive wish for omnipotence and control over her consciousness and unconsciousness, as well as materials and persons involved in the research. This is not to imply that there isn't great value in working reflexively and mulling over our motivations for selecting our research topics and interpreting our data in a particular way – quite the opposite. However, both the feminist identity checklist and the reflexive sociological approach can be taken up in facile ways that do not do justice to the complexity of the tasks they undertake, and further, these approaches assume that our decisions are rational and fully conscious. If combined with a psychoanalytic sensibility, these strategies can go much further to consider the irrational, affective, intrapsychic experience of research.

Geographer Felicity Callard elucidates why psychoanalytic concepts like abjection and the ego are enthusiastically embraced within geographical analyses of space and, I would add, the social sciences more generally, while other concepts like the death drive and repetition compulsion are not.[42] Callard argues that the former concepts are easily domesticated and assimilated into "models of resistance, agency, and resignification"[43] common to a social constructionist approach. To do this is to bypass what is arguably psychoanalysis' greatest discovery and insight: the unconscious.

I would add that concepts like the ego and abjection are also over-used within the social sciences because they can be assimilated into surface imagination cultures that value the dramatic transformations described by Callard, who understands psychoanalysis to be *incommensurable* with other theories of socio-cultural formation like social constructionism.[44] Further, a positivistic approach and a psychoanalytic approach are utterly irreconcilable.[45] Psychoanalysis is appealing because its theories offer possibilities to think through the psychical aspects of socio-cultural life in a way that honours the intimate, individual experience within the social. Mary Thomas asserts that "for feminist research to be politically useful might require a loosened grip on the logical world and a consideration of the seemingly illogical, the unspeakable, the deniable, and the invisible connections between social action and psychic life."[46] I am grappling with how to represent the stories that seven women have shared with me about their bodies and their cosmetic surgeries. A social explanation of these stories would encompass only part of their lives and exclude the important affective, irrational experiences that are a part of their engagement with cosmetic surgery.

Psychoanalytic analyses are sometimes critiqued by social scientists because they are difficult or impossible to verify, which compromises the validity of the research. Qualitative researchers committed to feminism and anti-oppression have made critical interventions into research by re-casting the research project as collaborative and co-created by the researcher and interviewees. One technique often used by qualitative researchers using interviews is to check that their analysis correlates with the interviewee's analysis, and if there is agreement the analysis is deemed to be an acceptable one. A potential danger of this idealized vision is that both the researcher and the interviewees are taken as fully rational subjects who are able to logically consider interview texts to produce a definitive truth in their analysis. This approach can also be manipulated by a researcher who presupposes in advance that the interviewees will probably agree to her analysis of the research data. It is more common for the researcher to report correlating her findings with the interviewees' analyses,[47] but it is far rarer to find examples of researchers working through a disagreement when using this method of validating analyses. Many researchers use this approach only when it is "safe." Checking with interviewees can be a means of disavowing that *all* analyses of interviews are necessarily interpretive[48] and infused with the researcher's emotional, intellectual, and political attachments, and instead shores up positivist hope for a pure knowledge gained by observation. This is not to say that as researchers we ought to be able to write about others with impunity, or that it is worthless to make research findings accessible; rather, this method of verifying research findings is often used uncritically and has the potential for disingenuousness. Certainly for community-based, collaborative, and action research projects, it is crucial for researchers to consult with participants about their analyses, to ensure that the findings are meaningful to the communities that the research seeks to record stories about. Further, if the analysis does not coincide with the interpretation of the research participants, it is important to consider seriously why this may be, as well as the consequences of competing analyses. Indeed, engaging with opposing interpretations of interview data can enrich the analysis and bring the research to life for the reader in a way that a one-to-one correspondence of interviewer and interviewee analyses cannot.

Approaching from Psychoanalysis

For a psychoanalytically informed researcher, it is important to distinguish between *psychoanalysis* and a *psychoanalytic approach to research*. *Psychoanalysis* is the process of undergoing a therapeutic analysis with a trained analyst who has undergone and completed an analysis as a component of their psychoanalytic training. A traditional analysis typically involves meeting three to five times a week over the course of several years. Thus, a relationship develops between analyst and analysand through which they can determine the course of treatment together based upon a deep and developing understanding of the analysand's history and present. In contrast, a *psychoanalytic approach to research* is a theoretical and ethical position that posits first and foremost an unconscious component to individual, social, and cultural life. A researcher using a psychoanalytic approach may or may not be a trained analyst, and may employ a particular theoretical approach in their work (e.g., Freudian, Lacanian, Kleinian, and so on) or a combination of these perspectives. Most frequently, psychoanalytic researchers study cultural texts and products as a channel to negotiate the complicated ethical impasses that might arise from conducting qualitative research with human participants.

Interviews undertaken from a psychoanalytic perspective occur in a very different context from the inter- and intra-subjective exchanges of talk in psychoanalysis. Often, researchers meet with the interviewees once or twice, and the interviews are conducted according to the questions and topics that are determined by the researcher. A therapeutic result is not identified as an objective for the research interview because there is not enough of a relationship to foster therapy, many psychoanalytic researchers are not trained as analysts, and it is not appropriate to conflate the aims of therapy and research. Instead, the researcher's focus is directed toward their own responses to the interview and the interviewee (especially strong emotions like boredom, anger, love, or irritation), and the interview story is treated as a cultural text for interpretation. A particular advantage of this approach is that the researcher is able to think more deeply about the absences, gaps, and leaps of logic within the interview story.

By using psychoanalytic theory to inspire research methodology, an analysis that considers the strictly social aspects of subject formation is moved in the direction of thinking about how the individual and the particular are formed psychically and in relation to others. As such, the participant in psychoanalytically informed research ought to be distinguished from the subject of positivist study in two important ways. First, the participant in psychoanalytically informed research is assumed to be non-rational and non-unitary. Premised on a particular ontological theory of the subject, this perspective recognizes the role of the unconscious in social and psychic life in addition to the importance of intrapsychic conflict.[49] Second, the participant in psychoanalytically informed research is not expected to be able to narrate their life completely or speak an absolute truth. This methodological approach acknowledges and embraces the ineffable, emotional content of our lives that cannot be fully held by the surface imagination demands of positivist discourse. It also recognizes that when we speak, we convey more than we intend. One benefit of this approach is that as we acknowledge that there is more to the participant than their rational, chronological explanations of their life, we become more open to the illogical facets of life that do not make sense according to a conscious logic. Building on other ways of approaching qualitative research in the social sciences and humanities, we no longer feel pressed to offer an artificial closure to interview narratives, smooth over discrepancies in the interview story, or hold on to the fantasy of research ending in solid answers. Instead, we can think about the complicated questions that arise when we involve other voices in our research, and consider research as raising more questions than it answers.

In psychoanalytically informed research, the self is considered to be the "primary instrument of inquiry,"[50] a phrase that acknowledges the researcher's subjectivity and also their agency in interpreting fieldwork data. Considering the researcher an instrument of research calls for particular attention to the intrapsychic facets of research, so that the researcher can acknowledge their emotional conflicts and attachments to the field. The researcher is obligated to pay attention to moments of friction and it is assumed that every field of research is likely to provoke emotional conflict in the researcher (conflicts that are both unforeseen and predictable).[51] Their choice of research topic and setting in particular is conceived of as structured not only by a rational decision but also by inner subtleties and unconscious dynamics.[52] Thus, this approach rejects the rational, complete modern subject as well as the modernist belief in progress over the course of history, opening up the research project and analysis of narrative to examination that holds the synchronous and diachronous elements of psychic experience.

In addition to conducting interviews, participant observation, and other kinds of fieldwork, research that employs a psychoanalytically informed methodology collects other forms of data. Because intrapsychic dimensions are critical to understanding the construction of the research, the researcher's dreams, jokes, parapraxes, and fantasies are conceptualized as data.[53] This data is used to understand how the researcher's subjectivity, identifications, and transferences structure the present fieldwork. Recording field notes and post-interview reflections becomes a matter of critical importance, rather than a prosthetic device of the transcript and the researcher's memory. The notes should include not only material on the physical reality of the interview or parts of the interview that were not recorded on tape but also the researcher's emotions and thoughts in relation to the interviewee as well as the space in which the interview is conducted. Because we are not psychoanalyzing the research participant[54] and therefore cannot interpret intrapsychic and intersubjective experiences from their perspective, all we have are our own intrapsychic processes (transference, identification) and these field notes can be incorporated into the interview story as clues for the researcher.

Each of the interviews I conducted for this research is unique and raises its own questions about surface imagination fantasies in contemporary cosmetic surgery practice. The interviews ranged in length from forty-five minutes to one hour and thirty minutes, and took place in the interviewees' homes (Tigerlily, Melinda, Tonya, Nicanor, and Diana), a university office (Victoria), and a tea room (Leah). My analysis of the interviews originates from the methodological perspective of grounded theory,[55] analysing the transcripts and my field notes in relation to each other in order to identify patterns and themes, rather than attempting to link the interviews with a pre-established theoretical framework and literature. A grounded theory approach allows the researcher to develop themes organically and to be open to unexpected interpretations offered by interviewees. Connecting a grounded theory approach to interview analysis with my development of a psychoanalytically informed method of poetic transcription offers the reader a unique and creative context for understanding interview transcripts.

John Shostak understands the inter-view as an open process that generates an intersubjective and intertextual commitment between the researcher and an other (the participant) which then serves as a foundation for ethical engagement between researcher and research participants. By cleaving the word in two – inter-view – Shostak proposes a reconsideration of a practice of speech (interviewing) that is pervasive in North America through talk shows, hiring procedures, market research, and sales, not to mention our contact with professions such as medicine, law, and policing.[56] This fissure in the word inter-view compels us to think more deeply about the seeing that happens between people when research interpellates the research participants' lives.

A psychoanalytic approach presupposes that there is a psychic rupture or trauma that is unique to each individual, that this rupture is unconscious, and that it structures one's life experiences.[57] In order to think about the interview psychoanalytically, the researcher must take the unconscious seriously. However, the researcher is very limited in how they might do this due to the limitations of doing research in a non-therapeutic setting. One starting point might be to think of the interview vis-à-vis Jacques Lacan's warnings about coming to an understanding hastily, when he says that "to read does not obligate one to understand. First it is necessary to read ... avoid understanding too quickly."[58] In this way the interviewer takes seriously the singularity of the interviewee's experience. They might think about the unconscious as it relates to the social or they might offer an interpretation of interview data that resists closure since the researcher cannot comment on the interviewee's unconscious due to the fact that this interview happens outside the analytic relationship.

In this endeavour of thinking about the unconscious as important, we are confronted with the idea of a psyche that is "deeply antagonistic to change [as well as the possibility of] the individual trapped in the repetition, rather than the suppression of traumatic formations; and deeply rooted, unsmiling fantasies."[59] The unconscious is not a "cultural artefact"[60] and it cannot be resignified at will. In Jean Laplanche's words, the unconscious is "not a stored memory or representation" but rather a trace, "a waste-product of certain processes of memorization."[61] In "The Ego and the Id" (1923) Freud explains that the role of the ego is to act as a mediating space between the unconscious (id) and the preconscious-conscious (perception-consciousness system and the external world), and he describes the ego as "a poor creature owing service to three masters and consequently menaced by three dangers: from the external world, from the libido of the id, and from the severity of the superego."[62] There is no way of gaining unmediated access to the unconscious (nor would we want to!); however, because "repression is never entirely contained or complete,"[63] we can say that the unconscious (signifier) erupts onto the scene through jokes, slips of the tongue, and the parts of the story that don't quite seem to fit together. The ego is at the level of surface imagination: a mediator attempting to construct a narrative of the self that positions the individual as heroine or victim, without nuance, and fully held together.

While psychoanalytically informed researchers cannot psychoanalyse individuals or offer an analysis of "*personalized* unconscious libidinal workings,"[64] they can use qualitative interview research to put forward an ontological theory of subjectivity that complicates notions of identity to include what cannot be said or observed.[65] In *The Colonization of Psychic Space: A Psychoanalytic Social Theory of Oppression*, Kelly Oliver argues that accounting for the unconscious is an ethical gesture that recognizes that since we are not "transparent" to ourselves, we cannot see others "transparently," so all we can do is engage in the act of interpretation and question our motivations and desires.[66] Oliver's appeal to researchers to think of continual questioning and interpretation as an ethical response to the unknowable, unconscious kernel within our experience guides me toward thinking deeply about how my interview narratives are re-presented in my research.

The transcript is like a photograph in that it fixes the interviewee's life into the stillness of text: the moment of the interview's time becomes the total representation of the interviewee. Shostak phrases it beautifully when he says that "a narrative kills ... the profile is transfixed, borrowing its life from the interpretations made by others, haunting intertextually, later writings and readings."[67] The transcript itself is likely not a closed, linear product, but the demands to present definitive answers and conclusions in presentations, papers, and grant proposals can tempt the researcher to try to do so. Shostak compares this process of managing the transcript in research to Lacan's notion that language destroys by substituting the dead, indifferent concept for the vivacity of life.[68] This inevitability requires researchers to approach the reading of transcripts and re-presenting them in research carefully and thoughtfully. Shostak cautions the researcher against deadening the interview through trying to fill in the absences that are present in transcripts. He evokes Lacan's story of coming across a tablet of ancient hieroglyphics in the desert: encountering this tablet confronts us with the wholly symbolic character of language. While we are utterly incapable of translating or understanding the hieroglyphics of the tablet without other information, we are capable of discerning that the hieroglyphics are signifiers that hold meaning.

Shostak cautions that the interviewer, when encountering the interview, is at a disadvantage compared with an encounter with hieroglyphics since, in the former case, the interviewer is unfortunately "all too familiar with the other who speaks."[69] In the interview, the interviewer is confronted with the everyday interpretive act of language, so it is critical for the interviewer to hold together the familiarity with the language of her transcript with the feeling of alienation produced by the hieroglyphics. Shostak also poses several new questions that we might ask of the interview transcript, including examining the text for its master signifiers;[70] exploring the range of subject positions and desires described by the interviewee;[71] considering how the interviewee regulates her speech,[72] arranges and distributes resources,[73] and understands the possibilities for action;[74] and how experiences are realized for the interviewee.[75] Asking questions such as these gives us new information that can be useful in representing the interview transcript.

Researchers commonly incorporate extensive quotations directly from the interview transcripts as a strategy for validating their interpretations. I decided not to employ this as my sole method for representing the interview transcript in this book for two reasons. First, the transcript itself contains many interpretive moves and decisions, which can be obscured by extensive quotation. And second, in reflecting on my own past research practice, I see the strategy of quoting extensively as one that defends against the anxieties generated from interpreting others' words and lives as they are offered through the interview encounter. So, in order to destabilize a conventional strategy of presenting extensive portions of transcript in order to accurately represent the interview narrative, I employ possibilities inspired by poetry and creative non-fiction writing. I read a great deal of science and nature creative non-fiction, and I admire two things in particular about this body of literature. First, many of these books are written from the perspective of non-specialists (and even nonscientists) for people who, like the authors, are interested in the topic because it is fascinating. This position of curiosity and marvel at the world, as well as the desire to communicate the stories of these wonders, is an admirable position for scholarship to hold. And second, creative science non-fiction is often truly interdisciplinary, where writers craft a narrative about a world that is outside of their own training and comfort. What happens in this interdisciplinary collaboration is that storytelling skills are employed to talk about subjects often considered outside the realm of storytelling. My processes of interviewing and transcription are opened up to critique, challenge, and analysis, along with a central tenet of my research practice, which is that story is central to human life and the process of living.

In the introduction to *Inside Interviewing*, James A. Holstein and Jaber F. Gubrium discuss Laurel Richardson's use of poetry as a textual device to represent interviews. They comment that poetry possesses a unique capability of representing that a text has meaning, but that this text can fashion meaning as well.[76] In addition to this important cultural function, poetry is often used when trying to communicate the unspeakable, or that which is too much to be held by words.[77] These two abilities of poetry are highly appealing to me as a researcher who is working with interview narratives about interviewees' relationships to their bodies and their experience of cosmetic surgery in a surface imagination culture. Poetry offers the researcher an expressive medium with which to witness the interview narratives, particularly when they appear senseless and filled with ellipses and absences. And finally, poetry experiments with the visual component of language, offering many different visual textual methods of placing the interview transcript onto the page.

Poetic Transcription

The style of representation that I employ to include portions of the transcript-as-object – for example, in "Grandmother and Mother" in "Making Introductions" – is referred to variously as poetic representation,[78] ethnographic poetry,[79] and poetic transcription.[80] I prefer the latter term, used by Corrine Glesne. Poetic transcription is the crafting of "poem-like pieces" using the participants' own words as the raw material.[81] The researcher's hope in using poetic transcription is to convey the affective content of the participant's responses to interview questions, to offer the reader some insight into the rhythm and tone of the participant's speech, and to distil the content of the participant's responses into its essence.[82] Glesne argues that the product of poetic transcription is a "third voice"[83] that is a mingling together of the participant's words and the researcher's representational practice.

In this book, poetic transcription is a psychoanalytically informed representational method that demands the reader pay attention to the interviewee's words, rather than skim through them quickly to get to the analysis. There are many reasons why the interviewee's words may fade into the background in academic writing. The most obvious reason is that the oscillation between informal interview talk and formal academic writing sets up a hierarchical textual structure, positioning the interview talk as decoration for the real stuff. The informal interview talk is assumed not to hold the same epistemic authority as the academic analysis of it, and thus can be more easily dismissed. Another reason for the fading of the interviewee's words is that it can sometimes be difficult for the reader to switch back and forth between different modalities of writing. A scholarly analysis is often invested in paying close attention to chronology and consistency of story in order to identify and discuss thematic commonalities, and contextualizes the interviews within a larger framework of scholarship. An interview transcript can leap across time and place, be inconsistent, and appear as though the knowledge that the interviewee expressed is self-evident because it is stated in a conversational tone. We use different skills when we read about research and when we have a conversation, so perhaps flipping between analysis and interview transcript effects a cognitive dissonance for the reader. Nevertheless, both readers and writers of research are interested in interviews precisely because they offer a perspective on knowledge and a fleshiness to the research that would otherwise be absent.

I am drawn to poetic transcription for a variety of reasons. Through them, I hope that the reader experiences more of the mood and meaning of each interview story. I hope the poetic transcriptions trip up the reader, causing them to stumble across the interviewee's words, unable to recover seamlessly to move on to the next paragraph. My appreciation for this style of transcript representation dovetails with Glesne's observation that when we as researchers experiment with form, we become more attentive to the intersubjective aspects of presenting the findings of our research.[84] In *Becoming a Qualitative Researcher*, Glesne outlines the five motives Eisner offers to explain why researchers might explore alternative ways to represent interview transcripts:

1   To generate compassion and understanding for the interviewee;
2   To emphasize the interviewee's singularity;
3   To encourage insight into and concentration on the intricacies of the interview;
4   To allow new questions to proliferate as the researcher explores the possibilities of a new genre;
5   To develop and expand the available representational resources of the researcher.[85]

These motives attend to the oft-neglected affective dimensions of research that I argue a psychoanalytic methodology can address. Poetic transcription is a direct challenge to a positivistic approach focused on categorization and generalization, and instead attends to what we might learn from the affective and the particular. Writing experimentation such as poetic transcription "helps to heal wounds of scientific categorization and technological dehumanization," according to Glesne.[86] I think a principal way poetic transcription can effect this healing is through its responsiveness to the absences and gaps in language and story, absences and gaps that are denied by surface imagination fantasies. Poetic transcription performs the same task as more conventional approaches to writing up the results of research by including exemplary quotations from the transcripts in order to distill them into representative fragments. Re-presenting an interview transcript as a poetic transcription encourages the reader to make her own interpretive decisions about what the interviewee is saying, rather than accepting the researcher's analysis as definitive. Further, poetic transcription highlights that the life stories that are told in an interview are not identical to the lives themselves, but are instead narratives or interpretations that the researcher labours to represent.[87]

My approach to poetic transcription is deeply indebted to, and inspired by, Glesne's work in "'That Rare Feeling': Re-presenting Research through Poetic Transcription." Prior to creating my poetic transcriptions, I coded the interview transcripts using a version of Barney Glaser and Anselm Strauss's constant comparative method to generate conceptual themes that recurred in all of the interviews.[88] When using this approach, the researcher must make interpretive decisions about where to discuss certain portions of transcript that might overlap across themes, and such decisions are often difficult. Glesne argues that poetic transcription aspires to demonstrate how pieces of the transcript narrative are connected to each other in thought and feeling.[89] The researcher uses the conventions of poetry (form and "concentrated language") to create a hybrid product that might not possess the literary sophistication of good poetry but allows the researcher a unique way of combining conceptual elements of the interview.[90] I found the rules that Glesne created to write her own poetic transcriptions highly useful:

1 The words come directly from the interviewee, not the researcher (the primary reason for this is elaborated in number 3 of this list);

2 Phrases may be taken from any point in the transcript;

3 When writing the poetic transcriptions, the researcher must keep in mind the interviewee's cadence of speaking and manner of phrasing. Thus, the researcher should try to preserve this through keeping "enough of her words together."[91]

As I will show in my explanation of how I crafted "The Gravity of Age," the degree to which I travelled around the transcript to pull out quotations varied greatly: sometimes I kept phrases in the exact order they appeared in the transcript, and sometimes I didn't. My extensive interview coding and organization was very useful for defining what I interpreted as essential features and themes of the interviews, and offered a solid foundation upon which to write the poetic transcriptions. I use the poetic transcriptions as a complement to a more conventional research writing approach, and I think that the co-existence of these genres strengthens the arguments that I make throughout the two chapters of interview analysis and contextualization.

I would like to turn now to a detailed explanation of how I wrote the poetic transcriptions, in the context of "The Gravity of Age," crafted from Tigerlily's transcript. Figure 1.1 on pages 38–9 shows the text taken directly from the original transcript (where I have highlighted in bold the parts of the transcript that I have used to create the poetic transcription) and the finished poetic transcription. Two frequently repeated ideas in Tigerlily's interview were that she had a "turkey neck" and that aging was a force comparable to gravity in its unavoidability and heaviness. When I listened to the cadence of her speech on the tape, her voice itself was punctuated with pauses and emphasis, and dropped in tone when discussing the inevitability of aging. When I transcribed the tape, I used a comma to mark a very short pause, an ellipsis to mark a pause lasting approximately one to two seconds, and for pauses beyond two seconds, I marked the approximate length of time in seconds. This was immensely helpful in writing the poetic transcriptions. The spirit in which Tigerlily told me about her experience with cosmetic surgery was very matter-of-fact. She said, "my experience has been, not been dramatic at all, it's been very you know, middle of the road, and ah, I think a lot of women, there will be a lot more drama attached to it." Thus I decided that it was important to keep the poetic transcription from Tigerlily's transcript succinct, just as our interview itself was brief, efficient, and to the point.

In writing the poetic transcription to describe what Tigerlily had told me about the type of cosmetic surgery she decided to have and the factors that she took into consideration when making her decision, I wanted to convey two major themes of this interview: first, that Tigerlily's experience of her aging face and neck took her by surprise, as if coming from a mysterious force; and second, that her face and neck did not project to the world how she felt inside. I did this by emphasizing the "strange things" that happen to the face gradually over time, the surprising nature

Original transcript
Interview A, Tigerlily, 30 April 2007

(Page 1)
R – 98 or 99, okay. Um, do you want to tell me a little bit about what kinds of surgery you decided to have?

T – Well my neck was looking more like a turkey's, and that bothered me a lot, my eyes were starting to get hooded, and what really bothered me probably from an appearance point of view was that everything, the gravity had set in **and I had this downward pull to my face** that in a relaxed mode, **I looked miserable ah, unhappy um, cross or sour,** you know, look which ...

R - ... right, right ...

T - ... **which did not reflect how I felt in the least** ...

(Page 2)
R – Right, right. And do you think, um, what sorts of factors do you think came into you um, making the decision to have cosmetic surgery.

T – It was, really, primarily, I did, I wanted to reflect to the outside world more of how I felt. Ah, also, I've always been ah, careful to present a, an attractive appearance. I wanted to be more attractive. I didn't want to look like a, a witch?

R – Right.

T – Not sure, because **as you age strange things ... happen [2–3 second pause] to your features,** as well as your body ...

R - ... right, right, right ...

 (Page 3–4)
T – **When my neck started going, and I was sixty,** I think, **every decade another thing** (laughter) starts becoming more prominent and my neck started going, and **I remember being very surprised because my parents didn't have ...**

R - ... oh really?

T - ... **as much of a turkey neck,** let's say. And **that really bothered me a lot,** more than baggy eyes, or but, but it, overall it was that appearance of being ah, unhappy, miserable that, that bothered me.

Poetic transcription
The Gravity of Age (Tigerlily)

As you age,
Strange things
happen
to your features.

That really bothered me a lot; every decade another thing.

When my neck started going,
I was sixty.
I remember being very surprised
Because my parents didn't have as much of a turkey neck.

The gravity had set in.

I had this
downward
pull
to my face. I looked miserable, unhappy, cross or sour.

Which did not reflect how I felt in the least.

1.1 Composing poetic transcriptions

of these changes (since they did not fit into Tigerlily's expectations), and the visual effects that the changes in Tigerlily's neck and face had on her appearance. I used the pauses in Tigerlily's talk to guide me in where to break up the line, and used her brevity of expression as inspiration to write short lines and stanzas interspersed with one-line stanzas that summarized her narration of her experiences.

The reader will note that I do not rely solely on poetic transcription when quoting from the interview transcripts. I also use a more conventional approach to representing interview transcript material, including quoting the interviewees within the text, as well as presenting block quotations for analysis. When I use a more conventional approach, I do so because the interviewee's narrative is presented in a straightforward and linear fashion, without contradictions in time or story. The poetic transcriptions are valuable when the interviewees narrate their cosmetic surgery in a way that conflates or collapses boundaries (especially temporal boundaries), or presents contradictory information. While I take responsibility for all of the interpretations presented in this book, when inconsistencies or narratives that do not follow a conscious, linear logic appear, I am most aware of my interpretive influence. The poetic transcriptions make these interpretations especially apparent to readers, and invite their own interpretations, especially when those interpretations are different from my own.

Conclusion

Modern cosmetic surgery has existed for over one hundred years in its current manifestation and practice.[92] While originally considered a part of the beauty profession, cosmetic surgeons toiled to elevate the cultural status of their occupation. They accomplished this feat by positioning their practice in the same realm as heroism and altruism and opened the field of cosmetic surgery to psychological and social questions. The profession disavows beauty as it also shores up cultural ideals of beauty through its practice. This is a perverse strategy that simultaneously accepts and rejects the social and personal role of beauty, which is conceptualized as negative and trivial due in part to the Cartesian ascendency of the mind. Within and without medicine, cosmetic surgeons have had to justify how their profession does not violate ethical obligations to not harm patients unnecessarily. Psychology has operated as a critical strategy for explaining how mental and emotional benefits offset the physical harm of surgical intervention.[93] Whether conceptualized as a medical intervention that rehabilitates the soldier back into his community and the workforce after war in 1914, or as a procedure that enhances the self-esteem and prospects for promotion of an office worker in 2014, the strategy of unhinging cosmetic surgery from beauty concerns has been extremely successful in making cosmetic surgery an acceptable option for many people, and in elevating the status of the cosmetic surgeon to that of an elite medical professional.

The language and ideas of cosmetic surgery enable us to imagine our bodies and the bodies of others as mutable flesh canvases; thus, it is critical to engage with the ideologies of cosmetic surgery in addition to the history of critiques of the practice. This is an unparalleled moment in history that promises to liberate our bodies from their contingencies, and also threatens to annihilate difference[94] in favour of a very narrow ideal that is white, thin, and Western.[95]

Cosmetic surgery can no longer be facilely analysed as patriarchal violence against women or as a result of airbrushed media representations of women. The problem with these kinds of analyses is that they consider cosmetic surgery as a force that impacts women from without in a unidirectional manner. It is important to be critical of the medical industry and its ideology that supports cosmetic surgery; however, this industry is not representative of those individuals who seek out and obtain surgery, or necessarily of those who perform it. This book is an inquiry into these narratives and what they can offer to a theory of feminine embodiment through the dermal and photographic surfaces. Complicating and opening up feminist understandings of cosmetic surgery, I use psychoanalytic theories in combination with social scientific methodologies to think about femininity in cosmetic surgery. These new understandings raise new questions about cosmetic surgery, particularly about the significance of surfaces, but also help to reframe the historical and cultural contexts within which cosmetic surgery has developed in the West.

FROM THE QUEST FOR RECOGNITION TO SURFACE IMAGINATION SURGERY

2

The interviewees in this study underwent their surgeries in contemporary North America. What are the historical and cultural conditions within which the profession developed and flourished in Europe and North America, and what are the resulting social and cultural understandings of cosmetic surgery? In particular, how has this context forged the important link between the embodied psychical surface of the skin and the topography of the photograph?

This chapter begins with an overview of modern cosmetic surgery as a medical specialty and cultural phenomenon, focusing specifically on the profession's quest for legitimacy and the gendered and racialized nuances within this commercialized field. In the section "The Quest for Recognition," I argue that the profession strategically emphasized the psychological outcomes of cosmetic surgery over the beauty outcomes in order to legitimate surgical interventions. Indeed, cosmetic surgery and psychoanalysis emerged in the same moment in history, and they have been entwined ever since. Dynamic power relations between surgeons and patients are a mixture of capitalist exchange and the entrenchment of body ideals in a sexist and white supremacist society. Furthermore, the relationship between doctors and patients is ambiguous because, in this medical encounter, unlike the majority in the West, the patient self-diagnoses. The relationship traverses into further murky waters as surgeons consciously and unconsciously develop their own signature styles, which are often justified by recourse to classical aesthetics and the history of Western art.[1]

Next, I turn to an analysis of contemporary cosmetic surgical cultures in the section "Pygmalions and Pragmatists." Drawing on Virginia Blum's important work on the pervasiveness of cosmetic surgery and surgical attitudes toward the body, I evaluate the cultural impact of understanding our bodies as the raw material of surgical alteration. I see three major shifts in contemporary cultural understandings of cosmetic surgery.[2] First, in the late nineteenth and early twentieth centuries, cosmetic surgery is understood as a secretive, deceptive, or suspicious pursuit, either because the desired outcomes are in the service of vanity or because they reflect a wish to camouflage or erase congenital, accidental, sexual, or racial difference. Second, from the mid-twentieth century until the 1980s, the move to project the desire to have cosmetic surgery onto larger-than-life celebrities propels the surgical act into the public realm. Celebrities exist as visual objects that give substance to new ways of thinking about the body's surface as transformable. We can maintain our moral outrage but still enjoy the plasticity of the body because we have no relationship to these figures outside their images. This is an important and gradual shift toward thinking about embodiment in a way informed by surface imagination. And third, in the late twentieth and early twenty-first centuries, ordinary people become the celebrities of surgical stories, coming onto the media scene with a surgical journey that is transformed into a story for the viewer's consumption and inspiration.

I address the makeover – a process in which an ordinary person becomes a celebrity, initially through glamorous hair, makeup, and clothing, and now through cosmetic surgery (called an "extreme makeover" on reality TV) – as a cultural moment that mobilizes surface imagination fantasies. The makeover is well positioned to incorporate cosmetic surgery into its fold because both use discourses of self-transformation and self-improvement through appearance. The extreme makeover highlights the pursuit of beauty as legitimate specifically on the grounds that the makeover candidates experience positive psychological effects through changing the body's surface, as I discuss in "Makeovers and Surfaces."

The scenography of the makeover hinges on one key element: the before and after photograph. Without this backdrop, the makeover cannot be staged. The before and after photograph operates as a device to fix the star of the makeover in time and space. In the before photograph, spectators are encouraged to see the tragedy and desolation in the face of the protagonist, assisted by bad fluorescent lighting, lack of facial expression, and a spoken monologue of personal tragedy. This singular piece of detritus from the previous passive life suggests that the protagonist's true life – which is, of course, an active life of happiness and acceptance – has not yet begun. In contrast, the after photograph depicts a happier, glossier, and improved protagonist, poised on the precipice of her new after life, complete with much better lighting. As cosmetic surgery stories become figured as makeover stories of overcoming and encountering loss,[3] the photograph is an important piece of evidence.

In the case of cosmetic surgery, photography is the medium through which the patient can compare her history to her present and imagine her future, although the photograph is not any of these points in her history, but rather a temporal messenger. Photography offers encouragement, shows what surgery can achieve in a surface imagination culture, and endorses and provides confirmation of transformation through digitally altered and/or before and after photographs. For cosmetic surgery recipients, before and after photographs become an autobiographical text that is often accompanied by a testimony of struggle and triumph over a persecutory and cruel body. Photography is a foundational medium in the construction of a surgical culture, and in "Photography and Loss," I explore the multifarious roles that photography inhabits in the psychical and social experiences of cosmetic surgery. It is important to think through the various functions of the photograph, since it is the idealized surface of cosmetic surgery to which the de-idealized surface of the skin is compared. Specifically, I consider the roles and implications of before and after photographs, including airbrushing and digital manipulation techniques, for cosmetic surgery.

The Quest for Recognition

The history of cosmetic surgery in North America exposes dominant cultural ideologies about the relationships between character and appearance and health and illness, as these connect with European ideas about science, race, and colonialism. Psychoanalysis has a parallel history to cosmetic surgery, since these two emerging professions explored common human problems and have buttressed each other's claims since their inception. Popular perceptions of cosmetic surgery shifted radically from the nineteenth to the twentieth centuries as a result of this relationship, as well as the effects of the First World War and an increasingly professionalized cosmetic surgery industry. Shedding its image as a practice to deceive others, the early twentieth-century cosmetic surgery industry engaged in a decades-long public relations campaign that touted its legitimate applications. These applications acknowledged and accepted the relationship between psychological well-being and physical appearance, and the relationship between the individual and the society. Contemporary North America can, therefore, be accurately described as a surface imagination culture in which we can all imagine modifying our bodies and the bodies of others through surgical intervention.

European philosophical ideas about the relationship between truth, beauty, health, and goodness continue to contribute to the positive valuation of beauty and negative valuation of ugliness. These ideas were crystallized in the science of physiognomy, which flourished from the seventeenth to the nineteenth centuries. Physiognomy is the scientific study of facial features for the purposes of determining moral character. Johann Caspar Lavater, pastor and author of *Essays on Physiognomy* (1775–78), expanded and popularized physiognomy, which gained ready acceptance in Europe due to the historical philosophical conceptions about the relationship between beauty and morality.[4]

In 1798, Pierre Joseph Desault gave the name "plastic" to surgery that aimed to change the appearance of the body.[5] These first modern operations restored function or appearance that had been lost due to circumstances of birth or accident, and relied largely on skin grafting.[6] Plastic surgery had as its aim the reshaping of the body and face, an action that was contraindicated by common Western religious and moral ideals, which were reinforced by the science of physiognomy. The development of plastic surgery generated many moral questions because it promised a permanent change to the so-called natural body. Surgery came to be seen as a disreputable profession whose goal was to conceal deformity or disease that, according to physiognomy and some Christian beliefs of the nineteenth century, were God's corporeal reprimand for sin.[7] Later, bearing the weight of a physical deformity with cheerfulness and good humour became a sign of good character and acceptance of God's will, as opposed to a divine punishment. By the nineteenth century, the development of the cosmetics and fashion industries in Europe and the United States heightened cultural anxieties about the potential for corrupt, criminal, or degenerate individuals, and particularly women, to conceal their inner selves from the world for personal and economic profit.

Modern nose surgery began to develop in the seventeenth century as a response to epidemic syphilis in Europe, but was not further pursued until the nineteenth century.[8] With the publication of Carl Ferdinand von Graefe's *Rhinoplastik* in 1818, this appearance-altering surgery became commonly known as plastic.[9] One of the symptoms of acquired or congenital syphilis was an infection of the bone and cartilage that resulted in a sunken nose (also called the "saddle nose deformity"). Surgeons experimented with paraffin injections, animal bone implants, and a technique called the pedicle flap in order to reconstruct the missing syphilitic nose.[10] Because of its complicity in concealing a divine indicator of depravity, public opinion roundly denounced plastic surgery as a disreputable profession.[11] Plastic surgeons, on the other hand, conceptualized their work as merciful because it assisted patients to pass as healthy by remedying their disgrace-tainted faces.[12] The association of the saddle nose defect with syphilis and immorality lasted well into the twentieth century in the United States.[13]

However, the nose is imbued not only with connotations of disease and sinful sexuality. The nose is also a site onto which racist European anxieties about racial and cultural difference are affixed, and the history of cosmetic surgery highlights this unease. Sander Gilman's *Making the Body Beautiful* takes the nose as its central object of study in developing the claim that cosmetic surgery was founded on the desire for "passing." Gilman argues that the recipients of aesthetic surgery are not pursuing invisibility – having one's appearance go unnoticed by the people in one's daily life. Rather, they are pursuing visibility, or passing as a member of the group within which one desires to be included (categories such as race, health, and youth).[14] The positive valuation of *passing as* can be fully realized only in visually oriented, surface imagination cultures; in discourses of passing, interiority is subordinated to exteriority. As rhinoplastic techniques were elaborated and improved upon in the treatment of the syphilitic nose in the nineteenth century, new techniques were developed that addressed the racialized nose as its subject. Following physiognomic logic and Enlightenment racial science, the nose that is too small, too big, too flat, or too short serves as a marker of individual and collective racial character.[15] Invoking the classical and medieval classification system of the Great Chain of Being, medicine and science created a biological hierarchy that justified scientific, economic, and social racism, as well as European colonization.[16] Depending on current trends in immigration and colonization, European and North American cosmetic surgery in the nineteenth century focused on the surgical assimilation of the Jewish nose,[17] the Irish nose,[18] the Oriental nose,[19] and the African nose[20] (in Gilman's terms). These so-called racial characteristics – whether or not they represented one's actual racial and ethnic heritage – were associated with being visible as within a specific racial category, and this legacy has permeated the history of cosmetic surgery.

In addition to significant developments in rhinoplasty and the coinage of the term "plastic surgery," the nineteenth century heralded two of the most important medical innovations for plastic surgery: anaesthesia in 1846 and antisepsis in 1867.[21] While these technologies are important to medicine and surgery in general, they are specifically vital to plastic surgery. In the pre-anaesthetic era, surgery was a last resort and highly traumatic for both patient and surgeon. The absence of anaesthesia made it difficult to think about surgery as a solution to even a life-threatening problem, and unthinkable as a solution to a problem with one's appearance. Further, the development of local anaesthesia by the 1880s eliminated the danger of dying under general anaesthesia.[22] With the patient's body and/or consciousness numbed by anaesthetic, the (plastic) surgeon could become more experimental and daring in the expansion of techniques. The discovery of antisepsis also made surgery a more appealing option, since it drastically reduced the formerly elevated chance that one might die of infection post-surgery.[23] These conditions, in conjunction with the First World War, advanced North American and European plastic surgery techniques. They also opened up debates about the legitimacy of plastic surgery and the distinction between cosmetic surgery and reconstructive surgery.

At the same time, developments were taking place in the new field of psychoanalysis, being articulated by Sigmund Freud. As Freud continued to theorize his discovery in his early work with hysterics, he articulated important connections about the relationship between psyche and soma.[24] Without the psychological motivation and explanation provided by psychoanalysis, cosmetic surgery could not have moved in the direction it did; it needed first to justify doing harm to bodies without a medical reason. The plastic surgeon needed to distance himself[25] from the negative label "beauty surgeon" which originated in the European renaissance and was put back into use in the 1840s.[26] The solution was found in the notion of happiness.

After the turn of the twentieth century, psychoanalysis was popularized in the United States as something glamorous, and its treatment of sexuality and the unknowability of the unconscious seemed almost magical.[27] Psychoanalysis and cosmetic surgery shared the common possibility and promise of complete transformation. Diverging from the majority of Western medical practices, these transformations are initiated at the insistence of the patient, who arrives at the clinic of the analyst or surgeon with a problem and therapeutic course that she has herself identified.[28] In *Creating Beauty to Cure the Soul*, Gilman argues that aesthetic surgery *is* psychotherapy,[29] since cosmetic surgeons cannot justify their practice without recourse to psychological explanations, particularly the pursuit of happiness. While it is a widespread misconception that the Hippocratic Oath instructs doctors to "do no harm,"[30] this phrase expresses a familiar understanding of the practice of medicine and surgery: that physicians and surgeons will act in the best interests of the patient and will not intentionally inflict injury or illness upon them. In order to circumvent the idea that cosmetic surgery is just a dilettantish wish for perfect beauty, surgeons used psychological explanations and concepts to justify their practice as a legitimate cure. The rise of surgical solutions to states of psychological distress happened at the turn of the twentieth century concurrently with a fashionable modification and spread of psychoanalytic ideas throughout the United States, a historical moment to which I return shortly.

Blum argues that psychoanalysis and cosmetic surgery share a parallel "cartography of the subject."[31] Cosmetic surgery borrows from psychoanalysis to justify its interventions into the body's surface, and psychoanalysis claims that symptoms on the body's surface are indicators of psychological processes. The logics of psychoanalysis and cosmetic surgery are consonant yet reversed in their speculations about the split between psyche and soma: psychoanalysis can cure the suffering caused by bodily symptoms through analysis, while cosmetic surgery can cure psychological suffering through surgery.[32] To complicate things further, Freud himself frequently used surgery as a metaphor for psychoanalysis: to convey the analyst's impartiality,[33] for the excavation of the unconscious,[34] as an intervention that must be brought to full completion,[35] and as a way to define the "analytic field," which, much like the "surgical field," can become contaminated (by the transference or the analysand's resistances, for example).[36] This metaphor justified the emphasis on the seriousness of psychosomatic illness and the analysts' profession. In turn, cosmetic surgeons reversed this logic into a psychosomatic explanation that positioned the beautiful body as a vessel of health and happiness.[37] Borrowing from Freud's assertion that hysterics suffer from being unable to put their experiences and symptoms into words, present-day cosmetic surgery asserts that a reliable indicator of a prospective patient's satisfaction is the ability to tell the story of her bodily suffering specifically and totally. If a patient is unable to be precise about this, she is more likely to return to the surgeon's office, unsatisfied and longing for more cosmetic surgery.[38]

Happiness becomes a goal of cosmetic surgery as surgeons appropriate psychological explanations and methods to justify surgery undertaken for purely aesthetic reasons. Beauty, happiness, and health are conceived as complementary: if one of these variables is removed, the others are likely to collapse. While those inside and outside the profession may critique cosmetic plastic surgery as trivial or bad surgery and view reconstructive plastic surgery as necessary and good surgery,[39] it is very difficult to delimit the boundary between reconstructive and cosmetic plastic surgery. One solution to this predicament is to reconceptualize disfigurement. The legitimate recipient of cosmetic surgery is seen as the victim of both accidental *and* natural disfigurement,[40] and a natural disfigurement is no longer understood as divine omen. Further, unhappiness is defined as a non-normative state, so cosmetic plastic surgery seeks to reconstruct the patient's happiness, a move that further blurs the difference between the cosmetic and the reconstructive.

The point is not to argue that surgeries categorized as reconstructive are unnecessary; accessing such surgeries has economic and social benefits for the patient. However, whether a surgery is categorized as reconstructive or cosmetic also has economic and social ramifications, as demonstrated in the example of breast augmentation for trans and non-trans women discussed at the end of chapter 4. A reconstructive surgery is likely to be covered under public or private health insurance, and there is little to no onus on the patient to justify the surgery to cosmetic surgeons as gatekeepers; the necessity of the surgery is taken for granted. The history of cosmetic surgery shows that the question of necessity is malleable and historically specific; a surgery that is classified as cosmetic may theoretically be as psychologically necessary for a patient as a surgery classified as reconstructive, and a surgery now understood as reconstructive may once have been considered purely cosmetic.[41] While the motivations for reconstructive surgeries are unquestioned and considered universally valid, surgeons and patients have long struggled to make an argument for surgeries considered to be purely cosmetic. Further, patients and surgeons continue to use psychological explanations to make a case for cosmetic surgeries since these explanations have proven effective.

During the first half of the twentieth century, cosmetic surgeons and the public turned to psychoanalysis and psychology to explain and validate the decision to undergo surgery for a purely aesthetic result. Here I examine four historical moments where psychoanalysis and (cosmetic) surgery come together to co-constitute one another: the Emma Eckstein incident, Karl Menninger's exploration of polysurgical addiction, Paul Schilder's concept of "body image," and Alfred Adler's "inferiority complex."

From 1895 to 1896, Freud collaborated with his colleague and friend Wilhelm Fliess in the treatment of Freud's hysterical patient Emma Eckstein. Fleiss operated on Freud and Eckstein in early 1895, and they received the same nose surgery on the turbinate bone as a part of their psychoanalytic treatment.[42] After the operation, Eckstein told Freud that she was in pain. Freud interpreted this as the formation of a hysterical symptom provoked by the surgical intervention, and was horrified to discover soon thereafter that she had developed an infection after a metre of gauze had been left inside her body.[43] This incident lead Freud to abandon the idea that physical intervention, from surgery to touching, should be a part of psychoanalytic treatment. In 1896, he moved away from his trauma theory – that patients experienced actual trauma to their bodies, particularly in childhood – toward the theory of the fantasy as the source of his patients' ailments.[44]

Karl Menninger is the first psychoanalyst to examine the psychical motivations for multiple surgeries in his 1934 article "Polysurgery and Polysurgical Addiction."[45] Menninger theorizes that surgery repeats the trauma of castration for the patient in a way that can be an "erotic capitalization," the fulfillment of the wish for a child, or the avoidance of something that the patient fears more intensely than surgery.[46] Menninger presents two case studies of cosmetic surgery patients (a labiaplasty and a rhinoplasty patient, to be specific) as examples of surgeries that do not fit into his theory because the recipients were made happy by their surgeries. What distinguishes these patients is that they obtain only one surgery and do not want more. For those who are obsessed with and objectify their malfunctioning bodies, psychoanalysis is a better treatment than surgery, according to Menninger.[47]

At the same time, Paul Schilder coins the term "body image" in his 1935 *Image and Appearance of the Human Body*, observing that the body is not just a biological entity or a perception, but is structured through "mental pictures and representations."[48] This means that bodies exist in the social and cultural contexts through which others interpret them, an idea that proved invaluable to feminist analyses of women's relationships to their bodies in the latter half of the twentieth century. This has also been a profitable idea for the cosmetic surgery industry, because it provides an explanatory model for a patient's desire to have cosmetic surgery: a patient wishes to make the image of the body that others see match the patient's image of the body. Gilman notes that Schilder's formulation of the body image places cosmetic surgery as an intervention that might alter the body image socially or physically. However, because the root problem is located in the mental image of the body, only psychoanalysis can fully address it.[49]

The final piece of this psychoanalytic puzzle is Alfred Adler's theory of an "inferiority complex."[50] The theory was developed at the turn of the century and became an invaluable explanatory device for cosmetic surgery by the 1920s. By the mid-twentieth century, the inferiority complex had become the most widely accepted justification for cosmetic surgery in North America. Initially, Adler was interested in the theory of organ inferiority, the idea that a physical weakness could become a site of psychological overcompensation. For example, a person who suffers from respiratory problems becomes an actor or a singer because they are so over-invested in their physical weakness that they overcompensate for it.[51] Cosmetic surgeons readily adopted this idea, claiming that an inferiority complex can originate in a physical feature and thus cosmetic surgery is a solution to the psychological problem of feeling inferior.[52]

During these moments of the intersecting histories of psychoanalysis and cosmetic surgery, analysts maintain Freud's conviction that working on the surface will not resolve the patient's psychical distress. At the same time, new and powerful ideas about the significance of the body's surface to psychical well-being emerge. The cosmetic surgery industry finds new ways to pathologize discontent with the body in order to present cosmetic surgery as a legitimate therapeutic cure. After the mid-twentieth century, psychoanalysis wanes in popularity in North America because its method, based on the presence of an unconscious, is not assimilable to surface imagination conceptualizations of subjectivity. Nevertheless, the histories of intersection provide insight into how cosmetic surgery became a therapeutic intervention structured by surface imagination promises that an operation on the body can resolve a patient's psychical distress.

While psychoanalysis became increasingly wary of physical intervention as psychotherapy, and cosmetic surgery conceived of its practice as physical psychotherapy, the professionalization of cosmetic surgeons, the rise of the mass beauty industry, and the First World War helped cosmetic surgeons create a powerful public relations campaign in the early to mid-twentieth century.

The disfigured soldier returning from the First World War radically changed social attitudes about disfigurement as a punishment doled out by God.[53] Surgeons now had a large number of casualties to experiment on in order to develop new techniques, and these techniques became the foundation of modern cosmetic surgery practice. The wounded soldier also opened up a new narrative for justifying cosmetic surgery that employed material and economic explanations. Because disfigurement caused by participation in combat was presumed to result in unemployment and therefore economic dependence, it compromised the returning soldier's masculine identity and dishonoured his contribution to nation.[54] As plastic surgery temporarily shifted its focus from operating on racialized facial features to reconstructing disfigurement inflicted by the ravages of warfare, the status of the plastic surgeon working at the level of appearance was elevated.

The 1921 founding of the American Association of Plastic Surgeons (AAPS), the first North American association of plastic surgeons, was a strategy to legitimize the practice by demarcating reasonable doctors from so-called quacks, although many of the reasonable, legitimate surgeons borrowed heavily from the techniques of quackery in the first quarter of the twentieth century.[55] Once plastic surgeons had a professional association, they attempted to cleave their field into two: the beauty surgeons, who operated on a purely commercial basis and without any regulations, and the plastic surgeons, who were highly skilled doctors and were required to follow strict guidelines established by their association.[56] By the 1920s, war surgery was effectively used to normalize cosmetic surgery in the public eye.[57]

During the Second World War, American women's magazines frequently published positive and enthusiastic articles about war surgery. While these articles were realistic in substance, their titles heralded the miraculous achievements of intrepid surgeons who saved soldiers from certain ostracism and unemployment at home.[58] This media coverage was strengthened by American cosmetic surgeons' willingness to use the media in their public relations campaigns.[59]

Haiken argues that as the Americans embraced a psychological world view after the Second World War, they were more inclined to seek private solutions to public problems.[60] American surgeons focused on developing their individual practices rather than influencing the direction of cosmetic surgery, while American patients criticized current beauty standards, yet felt it was more straightforward and less daunting to change themselves rather than challenge their society.[61] As the beauty industry amplified women's concerns about aging, cosmetic surgeons found a novel, individualized, and pervasive problem as well as the new audience they sought after the war to revitalize their practice.[62] Although surgery that focused on erasing race by operating on caricatured features had never vanished, post-Second World War cosmetic surgery in the United States saw an increase in Westernizing surgeries, particularly blepharoplasty (the creation of an eyelid fold performed specifically on people of Asian descent).[63] The popular media coverage of wartime cosmetic surgery established conditions for an enthusiastic, trusting, and optimistic reception of face-lifting, beginning in the 1950s and 1960s.[64] As face-lifting became a hot topic for American women's magazines, and increasingly affordable, surgery for beauty's sake launched the profession and culture of cosmetic surgery into the contemporary era.

Pygmalions and Pragmatists

The increased American interest in facelift surgery in the 1950s and 1960s marked a break from earlier ideas and a second turning point for the practice of cosmetic surgery into the realm of surface imagination. Unlike personal accidents or so-called abnormal features, aging happens to everyone who lives long enough. Thus, aging requires strategies that differ from those used to justify surgical intervention for accidental or congenital deformities. Instead, the body comes to be seen as a malleable flesh canvas and the individual is responsible for creating, revising, and maintaining the surface she presents to the world. Contemporary popular media do not often represent cosmetic surgeons as valiant heroes, as they did after the two world wars, but as artists and scientists. The artist and the scientist are no longer tethered to the burden of justification; they are committed to the pursuit of surface transformation. The makeover is important for both these new figures because it shares the transformational narrative of the surgeon-scientist's and surgeon-artist's work. The makeover story democratizes beauty, promising transformation for anyone. It is a product of surface imagination fantasies. In combination with tabloid stories about celebrity surgical makeovers, the surgical makeovers of ordinary people in reality television shows are useful as a device to justify everyday decisions to undergo cosmetic surgery.[65]

The conceptualization of aging as a pathological state after the Second World War opened up the field of cosmetic surgery in Canada and the United States. It moved from being a niche speciality serving only a few to one that can serve everyone and anyone. With the exception of the general practitioner, no other medical doctor can claim such a universal reach. The increase in face-lifting surgery in the 1950s was followed by what fashion magazines nicknamed the "Youthquake" in the 1960s,[66] a heightened interest in teenage culture and fashion that emphasized the beauty and freshness of youth. The 1960s also saw a slight rise in men's requests for facelifts, although this was a rare phenomenon.[67] While the popularity of cosmetic surgery increased from the 1950s onward, it remained a procedure that was done in secrecy.

In the late 1970s, a new kind of cosmetic surgery narrative began to surface in women's magazines: the story of the disastrous surgery performed by the incompetent or fraudulent surgeon preying on women's vulnerability to vanity.[68] These cautionary tales for women were about the high price paid for vanity, a precursor to the intense tabloid interest in the cosmetic surgery of the stars[69] and the rapid increase in demand for cosmetic surgery in the 1980s.[70] These warning narratives came full circle in the 1990s with the American scandal over the potential dangers of silicone breast implants. These more recent admonitory accounts emphasized that doctors and industrial manufacturers had been aware of the possibility of serious side effects such as silicone leakage and joint inflammation, and that patients received inadequate information prior to undergoing breast augmentation. The silicone implants scandal was further fuelled by a litigious American culture and great skepticism about the links between medicine and industry.[71]

In Canada and the United States, the majority of cosmetic surgeries now occur under what Davis calls the market model of medicine. In this model, the decision to undergo cosmetic surgery is framed by the "discourse of risk." The surgeon's responsibility is to offer the patient the most complete explanation possible of the risks and benefits of the surgery, so that the patient is able to give her full, informed consent to the procedure.[72] In contrast, the welfare model of medicine is framed within the "discourse of need."[73] What is important in this model is that the patient and surgeon completely articulate the reasons why the patient requires the surgery in order to justify the surgery to a state funding agency.[74] According to Davis, in the welfare model of medicine, cosmetic surgery is not a question of consumer choice but of exploring the motives and necessity for the surgery. Conversely, in the market model, the question of why the patient and surgeon deem the surgery to be necessary takes a back seat to offering the information that would allow the patient to make a good consumer choice in order to obtain the best value and result.

The majority of cosmetic surgery patients in Canada and the United States pay for their own treatment,[75] and the cost of surgery varies depending on surgeon and geographical location. As a result of competition between surgical specialties[76] and less demand and opportunity within the field of reconstructive plastic surgery, many highly skilled plastic surgeons turn to cosmetic surgery.[77] It is an appealing option for many reasons: surgeons operate on healthy patients with a high rate of satisfaction; there is a high turnover of patients, leading to greater economic profit;[78] and there are plenty of opportunities and challenges to develop as a surgeon. Thus, cosmetic surgery offers new plastic surgeons better material, economic, and career advancement opportunities. Patients are provided with a number of payment and financing options (including high interest credit cards that cater specifically to potential cosmetic surgery recipients), and the decision to undergo cosmetic surgery is framed as a consumer decision that balances the quality of the product with its cost. In the context of neoliberal medicine, physicians often dispense a commercial product[79] and the human body is treated like a work in progress, subject to current styles and functions, and a test site for the latest technology.

Blum argues that there is a process of "becoming surgical," in which the patient reconfigures her body according to the imagined gaze of the surgeon.[80] Envisioning the body's surface as fragmented and manipulable, in the way that the cosmetic surgery industry does, is key to surface imagination fantasies that locate identity and psyche at the level of skin. If the patient cannot explain her desires to the surgeon in a way that coincides with the current surface imagination discourse of cosmetic surgery, she will not be able to access surgery. Thus, the patient needs to know the cultural stories that circulate about cosmetic surgery, and particularly about cosmetic surgeons, in order to convince the surgeon.[81]

To understand how surgeons are represented in popular news media and women's magazines in Canada and the United States, I searched the *Toronto Star* and the *Globe and Mail* archival records from 1987 to 2007, as well as *Chatelaine, Harper's Bazaar, Vogue,* and *Cosmopolitan* for the same date ranges. The first two are newspapers that focus on Canadian national news coverage, *Chatelaine* is a major mainstream Canadian women's magazine that has been in existence for decades (since 1928), and the final three are major American women's magazines that represent a range in terms of writing and subject matter and are distributed globally. I decided to focus on the past twenty years in order to emphasize contemporary representations, rather than trace a genealogy. My method was to pull out the adjectives used by the authors and surgeons to discuss cosmetic surgery in order to identify how surgeons and observers narrated cosmetic surgical practice. In the process, I became aware of two specialties that received significant media attention in those twenty years: Designer Laser Vaginoplasty and cosmetic foot surgery. These two specialties allow me to illustrate the two major contemporary conceptualizations of the surgeon that I identified in the popular media stories more broadly: the surgeon-artist and the surgeon-scientist. To construct case studies of the surgeon-scientist and the surgeon-artist, I decided to focus on the websites of two American surgeons: Dr David Matlock and Dr Oliver Zong.

How do we think about cosmetic surgeons? What kinds of stories are intelligible within the discourses of cosmetic surgery? To answer these questions, I turn to popular women's magazines, newspapers, and websites advertising cosmetic foot surgery and Designer Laser Vaginoplasty. These cases are interesting not because they represent a horrifying extreme of cosmetic surgery or because they are particularly common but because they are practices that can develop only within a market model of medicine that responds to consumer demands. Further, these surgeries are publicly scrutinized in a manner similar to rhinoplasty and face-lifting in the early half of the twentieth century, and often labelled quackery. Finally, they are instructive because the methods used to justify them differ from a wholly psychological justification and extend the potential range of cosmetic surgery patients beyond those who can only explain their surgery in psychological terms. Studying these practices and popular press about cosmetic surgery demonstrates two new ways of conceptualizing the surgeon: as an artist and as a scientist.

NYC FootCare specializes in procedures such as foot narrowing, toe shortening, (big) toe straightening, and toe tucking (slimming of the pinky toe), which can all be combined with procedures that reduce pain such as bunion surgery: this combinatory approach is called the "foot facelift," and is NYC FootCare's specialty.[82] Cosmetic foot surgery is requested in order to enhance the appearance of the feet in high-heeled shoes and sandals through making the feet fit more comfortably into these shoes. Designer Laser Vaginoplasty is a trademarked set of procedures invented by Dr David L. Matlock, including the reduction and augmentation of the labia majora and minora, the reduction of the clitoral prepuce, liposuction of the mons pubis, and restructuring of the vaginal introitus and perineum for aesthetic reasons.[83] Designer Laser Vaginoplasty is requested for the purposes of giving the vulva a more youthful, symmetrical, and appealing appearance, according to Matlock's website.[84] Women bring high-heeled shoes and *Playboy* magazines into surgeon's offices, requesting to be moulded into the magazine or shoe's image.

The American Orthopedic Foot and Ankle Society released a position statement maintaining that cosmetic foot surgery "should not be considered in any circumstances and the Society does not condone its practice," and further, that "surgery should never be performed in the absence of pain, functional limitation or reduced quality of life."[85] Dr Vyta Senikas, the associate executive vice president of the Society of Obstetricians and Gynaecologists of Canada, has denounced the practice of "vaginal enhancement" surgery as yet another way of pathologizing women's bodies and elevating already high and unrealistic expectations of what women's bodies ought to look like.[86] In these position statements, professional medical associations make clear judgments on what constitutes legitimate and medically indicated surgery, and why cosmetic surgery of the foot, ankle, vagina, or vulva are illegitimate surgeries that do not fall within their mandates and membership. This distancing manoeuvre is a common feature in the history of cosmetic surgery. Legitimate surgeons and doctors are those who would never conduct surgery if pain, limitation, or an interference with quality of life were not present. These statements strongly privilege the physiological over the social and emotional and tacitly discourage the development of medical and surgical technologies for the sake of the technology itself or in pursuit of other human wishes (for beauty or conformity, for example). Contrarily, Dr Matlock defends the practice of Designer Laser Vaginoplasty as a valiant response to women's requests, asserting that women have the right to choose what happens to their bodies and to increased sexual pleasure (which he claims is a benefit of his surgeries), and he alternately uses scientific and artistic language to make these claims. Drs Zong and Tsentserensky do not make heroic claims in the written material on the NYC FootCare website, relying instead on understated scientific and pragmatic terminology: if the shoe doesn't fit, alter the foot through surgery so you can wear it, because we possess the technology to do so.

Articles about these cosmetic surgery procedures in popular women's magazines and newspapers reveal a great deal about how surface imagination cultures conceptualize the work of the cosmetic surgeon. As mentioned earlier, Blum tells us that in order for the patient to obtain cosmetic surgery and be satisfied with the result, she must visualize her body and face in the same terms as her surgeon.[87] Luckily, for those wishing to obtain surgery in Canada and the United States, the culture is steeped in references to the appropriate way to conceptualize one's body according to the surface imagination logic of cosmetic surgery. The vast cultural interest in cosmetic surgery builds on what Blum classifies as the "borrowed quality" of women's bodies,[88] which is the feeling that women never truly possess their bodies, let alone body parts that have been modified by the surgeon's scalpel or manufactured by a chemical company.[89]

One way in which the practice of cosmetic surgery is narrated is through language borrowed from artists and art history. Surgeons use aesthetics in order to justify surgical intervention and are compared to sculptors in popular media. The verbs that are used to talk about surgical technique evoke the artist's profession: the surgeon *carves* the flesh into a more pleasing shape,[90] the body is *contoured*,[91] liposuction becomes *liposculpting*,[92] and the face is *moulded*.[93] The descriptions of cosmetic surgery include statements of how the patient is offered "an individualized *palette* of choices,"[94] that one chooses a particular surgeon because one likes his "*work*,"[95] and that the goals of cosmetic surgery might include *symmetry*[96] and becoming more "*classically attractive*."[97] Magazine and newspaper articles about cosmetic surgery refer frequently to the history of European art, for example, justifying present ideals of breast size and shape by association with Renaissance painting,[98] comparing Michelangelo's marble sculpture of David with the cosmetic surgeon's flesh sculpture,[99] and even dubbing Dr Matlock the "Picasso of vaginas"[100] (an incongruous choice of artist, indeed!). These references to art and aesthetics are vague and either clichéd or uninformed.

Furthermore, they function to evade questions about racist and sexist surgical practice through recourse to a universal beauty, without acknowledging that this universal standard is particular to European art and aesthetic ideals and represents a political vision. By appealing to a lineage of beauty that stretches across thousands of years, the surgeon-artist can claim to be not merely catering to the trivia of vanity or whims of fashion but aspiring to the creation of a higher form of beauty. In the surgeon-artist narrative, the surgeon advocates for true beauty and is in search of aesthetic perfection, like Ovid's Pygmalion, the mythic character that sculpts Galatea in marble and whose wishes bring her to life. Blum notes that cosmetic surgery alters this myth in two ways: the surgeon works with flesh, not marble, and rather than transforming the art object into a living woman, the goal of cosmetic surgery is to transform the living woman into a photogenic object.[101]

Designer Laser Vaginoplasty serves as a case study in the surgeon-artist who transforms the raw material of the excessive, discoloured, and messy vulva into a tidy, unthreatening, and dainty organ previously attainable only through photographic airbrushing. According to Dr Matlock, women "want the skin to drape neatly over the clitoris," they want the "hyper-pigmented" tips of their labia minora removed to achieve "uniform coloration," and most of all they want perfect symmetry of their labia minora and majora, to remedy their profligate, aging, protruding, thin, or sagging vaginal lips.[102] Women are the "designers" who collaborate with the surgeon in order to shape their vulvas into a more "aesthetically appealing" product that they have chosen.[103] By referencing Western artistic practice and appropriating pro-choice discourse, the practitioner of Designer Laser Vaginoplasty evades being charged with promoting an agenda as well as questions that might arise from the fact that it is not H.W. Janson's *History of Art* textbook, but *Playboy* and other porno-graphic magazines that women bring with them to the cosmetic surgeon's office as reference material for their own "designer vaginas" (the common misnomer used in popular media for the process). While I share Simone Weil Davis's belief that "erotic tissue is far better enjoyed than removed,"[104] I also consider the justificatory apparatus that is used in the case of Designer Laser Vaginoplasty to be rather unremarkable in comparison to other cosmetic surgeries that use a common metaphor of the surgeon as artist.

Designer Laser Vaginoplasty garners a fair amount of media and feminist outrage. It clearly demonstrates the misogyny of the cosmetic surgery industry through its support of genital beauty standards that are largely created by pornography. However, my point is that this particu-lar case is remarkable only in perfectly encapsulating the surface imagi-nation metaphor of flesh sculpture, which privileges the aesthetic over psychological arguments for altering vulvas. Further, thinking of the sur-geon as an artist or sculptor acknowledges the surgeon's subjectivity and the possibility that a surgeon might have a particular style of nose or labia minora and majora (others have noted this fact upon examining the after pictures of other cosmetic surgeons[105]). Having an individual surgical style is held in tension with the appeal to a universal and timeless beauty. A surgeon might defend his individual style by appealing to universal beauty, but is more likely to deny a uniform application of a particular characteristic or technique in hisr work. The after photographs of surgical vulvas on Dr Matlock's website all bear a significant and disturbing resemblance to each other: while the before photographs show many common and delightful variations in terms of clitoral hood and labia size, shape, and colour, the after pictures share the same trimmed labia minora and clitoral hood that do not extend beyond the slightly plump (but not too plump, or protruding, or saggy) labia majora.

The second prominent depiction of the cosmetic surgeon is as a serious scientist, a pragmatist who understands the way the world is and works within this framework, rather than futilely attempting to change anything. This image too is an inheritance from cosmetic surgery's history of seeking public acceptance and legitimation. The theories of evolutionary psychology and sociobiology, popular in the media, now fuel scientific explanations for performing cosmetic surgery: evolutionarily, we respond to particular biological cues, so it is simply natural that some might want to alter their bodies to more closely emulate those cues. The correct proportions of the body and face can be determined mathematically; this is a shared legacy with the surgeon-artist's appeal to classical aesthetics. Technological expertise is emphasized in the image of the surgeon-scientist, who often perfects and builds on existing techniques to improve their cosmetic benefit. Nancy Etcoff's popular text *Survival of the Prettiest: The Science of Beauty* is one of many examples of television shows, magazine articles, and books that explain sexual difference and behaviour through biological and evolutionary arguments, usually oversimplified for popular consumption. This recourse to science is reminiscent of eighteenth-century physiognomy; however, the focus has shifted from what potential criminal traits lurk behind certain facial and bodily features to how our faces and bodies signal our potential for reproductive success. Beauty becomes a sign of reproductive health[106] and our responses and ideals of beauty are not determined culturally or rationally, but instead are simply "response[s] to physical urgency."[107]

A recent *Cosmopolitan* article that asks the pressing question, "Are Butts the New Boobs?" consults zoologist David Holmes to provide an explanation of why buttock implants could become a procedure as common as breast implants. Holmes's response is that humans' prehistoric ancestors were buttock-obsessed due to the strong links between buttocks and sex, and that this fixation led to an increase in buttock size that made heterosexual intercourse from behind more difficult. Thus, Holmes explains, heterosexual intercourse began to happen face-to-face and caused the consequent shift to breast obsession. He concludes that the increase in breast implants has led to the interest in buttock implants, since fake breasts do not trigger the same sexual response in men: so men return to "the original breast, the bum."[108] Holmes's response is both unoriginal (for example, Freud uses a similar analogy in *Civilization and Its Discontents* to explain the transition from smell to sight as the primary sense of sexual attraction) and also completely misconstrues evolution, which cannot possibly occur in the span of a generation or two (or the approximate length of time that breast augmentation has been a well-known surgical procedure in the West).

Not all depictions of the surgeon-scientist are as cavalier as Etcoff's – cosmetic surgeons are simply doing work in service of our innate biological desires – or the *Cosmopolitan* article on buttock implants. More commonly, the surgeon-scientist is depicted as a doctor with technological expertise and a desire to experiment with new techniques that cater to the public's wishes. In a *Globe and Mail* article, Dr Andrew Ress says about cosmetic hand surgery, "I was studying the functional things, tendons, muscles, and realized that no one had addressed the cosmetic issues and I began to think of the different ways to handle cosmetic hand surgery."[109] Cosmetic foot surgery is another example of surface imagination discourse that demonstrates the surgeon-scientist's commitment to both practicality and scientific discovery. Dr Zong, who coined the term "foot facelift," has been widely consulted by popular media to explain cosmetic foot surgery. The majority of the media coverage of cosmetic foot surgery walks the line between open contempt for the practice and tongue-in-cheek commentary. The standard formula is to begin with a discussion of common podiatric surgeries for conditions such as bunions, hammertoes, and corns (foot surgeries that are presumably acceptable and understandable) and then move on to discuss how Zong has experimented with these surgeries to improve the cosmetic benefit, so that now various techniques are performed for a solely cosmetic outcome.

Zong's online pamphlet "The Pinky Toe Tuck" reads like a fashion magazine, encouraging women to "consider a designer pinky toe that is as elegant as the shoes that will adorn them (*sic*)."[110] In a non-threatening, matter-of-fact manner, the pamphlet describes the procedure of removing bone and flesh from the pinky toe and emphasizes the freedom to wear any high-heeled shoe or sandal without the discomfort of the pinky toe's natural curvature. The pamphlet espouses the aesthetic and practical benefits of a pinky toe tuck, casually adding that, "as an added bonus the pain is also gone."[111] This copy is juxtaposed with x-ray pictures of women's feet before and after the pinky toe tuck, and the captions below each picture differ greatly from the kicky and casual tone of the rest of the pamphlet. "This preoperative foot x-ray is of a 25 year-old female who works as a legal secretary in a law firm. She has been wearing high heels since she was 18 years old. Notice how the 4th and 5th toe bones are bent," is the caption for the before x-ray. This is followed by the caption for the after x-ray: "This postoperative foot x-ray reveals the bony straightening associated with the pinky toe tuck procedure as well as straightening of the 4th toe bone."[112] This caption is markedly different from the pamphlet's copy: "The procedure is very popular in the winter months here in New York City since patients are easily able to wear their Ugg boots during the healing phase and then transform into their stylish heels for spring."[113] The linking of the confidante tone of fashion magazine writers – who possess inside knowledge of current brands and trends in fashion – with the authoritative voice of the captions is a powerful combination that gives patients a pragmatic and non-judgmental view of the practice of cosmetic foot surgery.

However, this view astonishingly elides the detail that high-heeled shoes often cause many of the problems that are addressed by cosmetic and other foot surgeries; instead, it asserts that scientific and technological breakthroughs can assist us to change our bodies according to contemporary fashion, since it is unrealistic to expect women to abandon fashion. The medical-scientific gaze into the body's interior offers sensible evidence for the cosmetic procedure, conjuring up the presence of x-rays in countless contemporary representations of medicine and surgery, and presenting the surgery in a familiar authoritative manner. The surgeon-scientist is not like the surgeon-artist since he is not appealing to a higher calling for beauty, but instead is responding to the material circumstances of women's lives through science and technology. However, both the artist-surgeon and the surgeon-scientist share the goal of transformation and both their narratives are critical to the unfolding of the surgical make-over story, to which I turn in the next section.

These narratives are linked to one another through surface imagina-tion: while aesthetic and scientific narrative devices are employed in their stories, they share a fantasy that transforming the body's surface will have a positive effect on the life of the patient. Because of this shared fantasy in the ideology and discourse of the cosmetic surgery industry, it does not matter which way the cosmetic surgeon's work is narrated, since the expected outcome of life transformation is the same. These are simply two strategies that can emerge within a surface imagination culture. The shared commitment to surface transformation is important to the un-folding justifications of cosmetic surgery practice.

Makeovers and Surfaces

In contemporary North America, the significance of the makeover to our surface imagination understandings of embodiment cannot be underesti-mated. The makeover story is almost exclusively gendered female and speaks to longing and hope for personal change. The makeover trope de-pends on the viewer identifying with the character's struggles and tri-umphs and thus a critical component is the notion that anyone can be made over. In movies, makeovers can help a character transcend class, overcome psychological difficulties, get ahead in the workplace, wow the high school, or get the man. Prior to the movie makeover (and, as we will see, the television cosmetic surgery makeover), the character is subject to the cruelty of others on the basis of her appearance. Nevertheless, she per-severes and is greatly rewarded by the makeover, which enables others to see her for the real woman that she is underneath. Elizabeth A. Ford and Deborah C. Mitchell call the moment that the character's true, beautiful self is revealed the "Cinderella moment,"[114] a glorious retribution for the character's often lifelong suffering and sometimes a revenge fantasy against those who perpetrated the past cruelty.[115]

However, the character must first submit to the makeover.[116] The con-temporary television makeover divides the body into pieces that are placed under the control of experts (specializing in hair, makeup, dress, body, etc.). This move is greatly influenced by surface imaginations that structure cosmetic surgery culture so that the body is divided into its component parts, which may then be individually altered for cosmetic, and thus psychical, benefit. While the before life of the ordinary person in television makeover shows is an interior life of complicated pain, the after life is a smooth, uncomplicated surface of a photograph or a series of brief filmed segments. These still and moving images chronicle the makeover recipient as finally content, doing everyday things shortly after her makeover, and revealing her makeover to friends and family during a party or other special occasion. Because they share the pursuit of beauty, acceptance, and change through a surface imagination perception that the real person can emerge through aesthetic modification, the makeover story and the cosmetic surgery story fit together seamlessly.

Davis distinguishes four features of cosmetic surgery that parallel the makeover story and highlight dimensions of surface imagination. The first is a before and an after: the decision to have cosmetic surgery marks a defining moment in one's life from which to examine the past and speculate on what the surgery will mean for the future.[117] As a time when one voluntarily gives up control for the purposes of self-transformation and self-care, the makeover is also a defining moment: usually the protagonist of the makeover story talks extensively about her commitments to family, work, or friends, which have left her with no time to care for herself. Here the interior life is problematic but the decision to undergo a makeover defines a refusal to be controlled by that interior, and a decision to control it through surface manipulation. Second, cosmetic surgery stories communicate a "trajectory of suffering": an aspect of the body hinders one's enjoyment and success in life, relationships, and work and thus causes great emotional pain.[118] This parallels the cruelty and hardship that the protagonist suffers prior to the makeover, and the inability of others to see beyond appearances; the subject of the makeover is thus a deserving one. In both cases, the decision to have cosmetic surgery or a makeover is a way of taking control over one's life and disrupting this trajectory by intervening on the terms by which one was cruelly victimized. Third, cosmetic surgery stories are often presented along with a series of "arguments and deliberations." That is, the women Davis interviewed anticipated potential negative reactions to their decisions, so they included the positive and negative aspects of cosmetic surgery in their portrayals.[119]

This aspect is not as readily identified in the makeover story. However, since the makeover requires the protagonist to surrender control for the duration of the makeover, in television makeover shows there are often small resistances, for example, to cutting hair or throwing away one's entire wardrobe. Finally, the key feature of cosmetic surgery stories is that they are about the individual's identity.[120] Like the division of one's life into a before and an after, the cosmetic surgery story retroactively reconstructs a life history to unify all the selves that are contained within the story. Inconsistencies and contradictions are negated under a unifying surface that imagines the self in an idealized manner. The makeover story also does this, and tells us that the true, radiant self is revealed through this transformation. It puts into the visual realm this resurfacing of the protagonist's identity.

The cosmetic surgeon's gaze is aesthetic and transformative, according to Blum,[121] and further, imposes a question on women in general: "Do you think you're attractive?"[122] Makeover and cosmetic surgery stories are highly individualized and focus on whether the individual feels she is attractive, rather than on the social, political, and cultural contexts that structure her feelings. Because the focus is personalized, the reality that the features under surgical consideration are those that are caricatured and racialized is erased and disavowed. As noted earlier in this chapter, cosmetic surgery in the nineteenth and early twentieth centuries explicitly addressed racialized features, and connected those features with negative social or personality traits. Cosmetic surgeons no longer describe procedures in this way; for example, while double eyelid fold surgery is almost always performed to transform an "Asian-looking" eye into a "Caucasian-looking" eye, both looks are described neutrally, as though patients simply have a personal preference for one over the other.[123] Thus, the ways in which racism structures very specific ideals of beauty is circumvented.

In her original study, Davis identifies that a central purpose of cosmetic surgery is to "becom[e] ordinary":[124] the women she interviewed want to move through their worlds unnoticed for their physical differences. The ordinary remains unexamined, just as the desired after of the makeover story does not question the gendered, racial, ethnic, sexual, and classed norms that make up the result. Another consequence of the focus on individual enhancement and becoming ordinary is that the makeover and cosmetic surgery stories gleam with middle-class notions of cleanliness and upkeep: as Blum points out, in the world of cosmetic surgery, you repair and maintain your face just as you would your middle-class house and garden.[125] Similarly, the makeover requires upkeep in terms of acquiring more products and clothing and maintaining and updating hairstyles. In cosmetic surgery practice, after an inaugural surgery, more surgery will be required to correct previous surgeries, maintain surgeries, or re-experience the satisfaction of the original surgery.[126] However, the constant maintenance required to keep up one's appearance is not featured in makeover or cosmetic surgery stories because, at the moment the protagonist is revealed as her true self, the story is over. Depicting the labour and expense of maintaining the after image would shatter the surface imagination fantasy, which presents the transformation as effortless and lasting: it is to be taken as a substantive internal change to the very essence of the transformed individual.

The makeover is a popular theme for reality television: the wardrobe in *What Not to Wear*, the hapless/hopeless straight man in *Queer Eye for the Straight Guy*, the car in *Pimp My Ride*, the body through cosmetic surgery in *Extreme Makeover*, the house in *Extreme Makeover: Home Edition*, or the plain, old-fashioned hair, makeup, and fashion makeover with a friend or family member in *A Makeover Story*. In 2004, Fox Television aired the controversial reality television makeover show *The Swan*. The premise of the show is grounded in Hans Christian Andersen's fable *The Ugly Duckling*, in which an ugly, clumsy grey bird is born in a duck's nest and does not resemble any of her siblings. The bird is mistreated and abandoned by the ducks due to her difference and eventually develops into a beautiful swan, a fact she discovers only when she looks into the water and gazes into her exquisite reflection. She joins a bevy of swans, and is described as the most beautiful because she is free of arrogance: it is her inner beauty that radiates outward.

In *The Swan*, sixteen women are given extensive makeovers by a team of experts over the course of three months, including cosmetic surgeons and dentists, a therapist, a life coach, and a personal trainer. Each episode chronicles the makeovers of two women. It begins with a synopsis of their life's suffering due to issues such as failed relationships, emotional abuse, and feeling humiliated by their faces and bodies. This focus on individual misery eclipses a social analysis of how factors such as classism, racism, and sexism have affected these women's lives. For example, many contestants on *The Swan* – like contestants on other cosmetic surgery reality television shows set in the United States, such as *Extreme Makeover* – did not have access to basic or adequate health care. As a result, surgeries like LASIK eye surgery and dental surgery were performed for their cosmetic benefits, yet in many cases alleviated the need for ongoing care (in the case of vision loss) and addressed the absence of care (in the case of dental care). After an intense segment that gives a rapid-fire and brutal account of everything that is wrong with the women's bodies and psyches, the viewer observes the women undergoing great emotional and physical stress over the course of three months due to surgery, malnutrition from severe dieting, physical exhaustion, and isolation from family and friends. At the end of the show, each woman's progress over the three months is assessed by the experts, and she gets the final treat: a look at herself, after she has been denied any kind of mirror over the course of the show, in a giant mirror that is draped in luxurious red velvet. The experts are presented in a highly visual manner through surface imagination means, as professionals whose compassion and expertise is apparent through their attractive appearance. They have white, straight teeth, bronzed skin, perfect makeup and hair, and wear lab coats, pantsuits, and skirt suits, all of which confer status and knowledge upon the experts (through referential status to professionalism and upper middle-class life). However, the episode does not stop there: the mirror gazing is only the penultimate event of the show. After both women have been revealed to themselves and the television audience, they are then pitted against each other and one is chosen to participate in the "Swan pageant," a beauty contest that serves as the season finale.

The visually climactic moment of any episode of *The Swan* is the reveal. I focus on the reveal because of its close affiliation with a surface imagination approach to identity in the cosmetic surgery makeover. As June Deery argues, the reveal exposes and exhibits the makeover subject to herself as well as the television audience.[127] Until this point, the show has guided the viewer through the harrowing experience of the women's transformations by sanitizing the surgical process; a series of fast-motion shots of the actual surgery and recovery turn the surgery itself into a magic trick.[128] One of the show's gimmicks is that the participants are forbidden from seeing themselves in any kind of reflective surface, and they are rigorously policed. In fact, most episodes depict a staff member rifling through the contestants' personal belongings immediately following her arrival on the set to ensure no contraband mirrors have been smuggled in. This absence of a reflective surface is sharply contrasted with the opulence of the mirror that the women gaze into during the reveal. The mirror is a ceiling-to-floor piece of glass draped in voluptuous red velvet tied back with gold cord, evoking the luxe décor of a fairy tale castle, or the red carpet entrance of celebrities attending the Academy Awards. While up until this point the show has focused on the unglamorous realities of the contestant's life (devoid of any gender, race, or class analysis), the reveal exists in the realm of fantasy and exteriority. Most of the women do not possess secondary or post-secondary education and are stuck in poorly paying jobs or unsatisfying marriages due to their socioeconomic class, race, and/or gender, but the reveal promises that their new surfaces will overcome these obstacles that are reconfigured as individual life choices.

As Laurie Ouellette and James Hay argue, the citizen of today is obligated to privately empower themselves,[129] and both the television makeover and cosmetic surgery take advantage of this obligation. In their words, the surface imagination conception of self is "a flexible commodity to be molded, packaged, reinvented, and sold."[130] When the contestant gazes at her image in the mirror, she is being introduced to herself as a product.[131] Nothing has changed for the contestant but her surface appearance, although lip service is paid to emotional and psychological work. Once they have completed the three-month-long ordeal, all the women look eerily alike since they share similarly augmented breasts, liposuctioned waists and buttocks, cheek and chin implants, hair extensions, stage makeup, false eyelashes, and bronzed skin. The reveal moment also masks – through its drama and glamour – the specificity of the beauty that is revealed, which is a white, middle-class, feminine beauty, particular to the current historical moment in the United States yet presented as universal through the contestants' uniform appearance and response to that appearance. They also share a response to that moment when they gaze into the mirror at their transformations: first they cover their faces and sometimes double over; express disbelief that they are looking at their own images while running their hands over their bodies and skin; and soon turn in every direction to get a better look at their bodies in a narcissistic display of acceptance. The contestants are frozen within the reveal moment. As the audience, we are supposed to suspend our knowledge of their social locations and histories and ignore their futures, which will necessitate a life-long commitment to cosmetic surgery to correct and maintain the procedures performed on *The Swan*. The reveal encourages us to bask in surface imagination fantasy along with the contestants and enjoy the spectacle of transformation as it is immobilized in time like a sculpture. As Jerslev argues, this body bears no marks of the surgical intervention and we may look at it from all angles (as we would the marble sculpture):[132] a surface with no interior, or a surface with a finally harmonious, happy interior is transparent to the outside.

Ouellette and Hay point out that as viewers of television makeover shows, we can occupy an array of positions in relation to the show's subjects:[133] we can identify with the subject's suffering, the experts' ability to give advice, or in many cases (particularly with regard to *The Swan*) we can assume the position of moral critic denouncing the superficiality of the transformation. *The Swan*'s reveal moment manipulates the ambiguity of audience identifications, because the camera directs our gaze as originating over the shoulder of the contestant. It also directs our attention toward the surface and imagistic qualities of the transformation, because the reveal moment is not about the psychological work the contestants have undergone,[134] but rather what has happened to the body on the skin's surface. We might imagine ourselves as the ugly duckling-cum-swan, gazing into our metamorphosed beauty (with either delight or horror at its generality) from this position; as the benevolent expert reaping the fruits of our labour through the contestant's delight; or we could take a voyeuristic gaze upon the mirror image. The mirror image is, in contrast to the photograph, a representation of the body that is generally reserved for the self. While the photographic image estranges us from ourselves because it can exist independently from the self in the public domain, the mirror image is unifying because it belongs to us. The formula of *The Swan*'s reveal sequence renders the mirror image public through the camera shot, encouraging the audience to voyeuristically take in the contestant's image as the contestant attempts to psychically integrate her made-over image. Through their initial refusal to see (covering their faces) and subsequent touching of their bodies, these women are attempting to take possession of their surgically produced skins. The interior of their body is finally at home in a beautiful exterior product. At the end of each episode, all the contestants possess a culturally valorized beauty that promises to improve their miserable lives through assimilation into an ideal that is structured by whiteness and middle-class-ness.

The Swan changes the makeover television show in the same way that cosmetic surgery has changed in recent years: it goes deeper beneath the skin's surface, in search of the interior, in order to transform its surface. Unlike the women in Kathy Davis's studies, the contestants on *The Swan* are not trying to become ordinary; on the contrary, according to conventional beauty standards, they are already average looking before the makeover and are trying to become beautiful and extraordinary as a way of coping with and overcoming the hardships and banality of their lives. The most fascinating feature about this show is that the transformations exist entirely on the surface. The women have apparently entered into the show's story line with many emotional, social, and psychological issues. While therapy and life coaching are provided, they are not the central foci of the show; the show pays only lip service to the psychological aspects of the women's lives. The centrepiece of *The Swan* is the implicit belief and message that altering the body's surface through cosmetic surgery can totally transform one's life. Blum accepts cosmetic surgery recipients' word that the emotional pain they feel is actually located on the surface of the body, and that sometimes cosmetic surgery does in fact heal: she says, "the surface of the body and the body image are where object relations, both good and bad, are transacted, not only in the formative moments of our identity, but throughout the life cycle."[135]

There was much outrage expressed in the popular media about this show. The criticism legitimately focused on the reinforcement of racist and sexist beauty ideals through potentially dangerous surgeries, the assumption that cosmetic surgery would heal the contestants' emotional lives (themselves structured by the violences of misogyny, racism, and/or poverty), and, of course, the beauty pageant as exploitative endpoint for the show. However, the most outrageous aspect of the show was ignored, which is the underlying claim that it is possible to repair our damaged psyches through altering our appearances, one of the oldest and most elided claims in cosmetic surgery's history. The makeover story is important to us precisely because it articulates the ways in which our bodies, faces, and skins can hold – and hence can possibly release – emotional trauma, a possibility that is generally unacknowledged both socially and medically. A critique of cosmetic surgery that only takes into account the ways that culture and society affect the outcomes of surgery cannot account for the ways that surgery might enable patients to work through difficult emotions, because the patient's wants are seen to originate from without. The contestants on *The Swan* rely on the revealing moment of looking into the mirror in order to see how their lives have changed, a moment that pinpoints and highlights how the image, reflection, or photograph is essential to the transformational stories of cosmetic surgery.

Photography and Loss

What indeed are nine-tenths of those facial maps called photographic portraits, but accurate landmarks and measurements for loving eyes and memories to deck with beauty and animate with expression, in perfect certainty, that the ground-plan is founded upon fact? (Elizabeth Eastlake, "Photography," 1857)[136]

As a tangible visual artifact, the photograph occupies the place of reminder, evidence, and promise within the culture of cosmetic surgery.[137] Although Elizabeth Eastlake's comments on photography are over one hundred and fifty years old, they express sentiments that many of us continue to hold about photographs as placeholders for memory that enjoy a certain authority as factual souvenirs of the past. The affective experience of poring over photographs is both deeply gratifying – as a comforting remembrance of a beloved – and at the same time fills us with longing. This is because the photograph eradicates its subject, condemning the subject forever to the instant of the shutter's closure as it comes to serve as the representative of the past subject in the world.

In a surface imagination culture, photographs are possibilities of what one might like to accomplish through cosmetic surgery, a source of inspiration, and the medium through which the patient can compare her history to her present, and imagine her future. Before and after photographs are transformed into self-contained visual autobiographies, often supplemented with a testimony of struggle and triumph over a tyranni-cal body.

Yet, the photograph is not the patient's history, her present, or her fu-ture, since it is dead. Timothy Don Adams observes that "autobiography and photography ... are equally haunted by the presence of the referent. Both appear to represent their subject in a strikingly unmediated fashion; both appear to reveal the real. Nevertheless, as forms of representation, both are not the subject itself but its imaging, reproductions of the refer-ent."[138] Furthermore, before and after photographs and malleable digital images serve as a support for the cosmetic surgical procedure and as ev-idence of its transformative value. However, in reality, photographs lie; they conceal more than they tell about what really happened. We say a photograph has been retouched, a verb that makes explicit the interfer-ence of the human hand upon the photograph's surface, the enhancement of colour, and the airbrushing of unwanted content. These alterations fur-ther distance the photograph's dead subject from the subject who lives on beyond this photographic cemetery.

As the medium of death and loss, photography fixes time into a per-manent image-trace. In contrast to the moving image, which through il-lusory movement sustains the fantasy and hope that the depicted subjects are alive, the stillness of the photograph impersonates death.[139] Photo-graphs have recorded some of the most traumatic moments in our recent collective human history, and also serve as reminders of trauma in our in-dividual histories. Jay Prosser describes the photograph as a "melancholic object" because it offers us a route to a past moment.[140] However, the ephemera that produced that moment are lost forever, making this an empty return that lacks the fantasized fullness of the half-moment between the photograph's birth and death. In his profound reflection on photog-raphy in the wake of his mother's death, Roland Barthes describes the ex-perience of looking at photographs as the "return of the dead."[141] That is, there is a transitory moment when gazing upon a photograph of oneself in which one is neither the subject nor the object of the photograph. Rather, one is *becoming* the object of the photograph, an object in general. In this moment of looking, one experiences a "micro-version of death,"[142] for death renders the living subject into an object forever. This experience is alienating; a strange and permanent effect of photography on the way we think about ourselves – structured by surface imagination – that contributes to the potential of viewing our bodies as surgical raw material.

There is another dimension to the photograph's occupation of an in-between space: it becomes the image and remnant of a person in a past moment, but it is haunted by its inability to fully hold our relationship to the person in the photograph due to its status as mere image. However, this feature should not be taken as a minimization of photographic images, for, as Susan Sontag reminds us, photographs are powerful: they can appropriate reality not just because they are an image-representation of a moment, but also because they are "also a trace, something directly stencilled off the real, like a footprint or a death mask."[143] A photograph appears to contain the real person within its narrow white borders behind a protective glossy window, so we continually return to it in search of that person. Eventually, we take leave of the photograph because ultimately it is an unsatisfying substitute. Photography shows us something that is no longer there, which is its first loss. The second loss, according to Régis Durand, is that no matter how long we scan the photograph, nothing "can lead back to its source – except precisely the sense of its having come from a source and of the ensuing transformation and loss."[144] Celia Lury writes that we have two options in the face of this loss: fantasy or fear,[145] or put another way, creating a story that will fill the loss or renouncing the loss altogether. Both options will come to fail us sooner or later.

Through photographs, we are faced with absence of the photograph's subject, and thus photography is an unconscious brush with death and loss. As an indication of death, photography illuminates loss in a way that allows us to begin to apprehend what has been lost.[146] A component of this apprehension is the use of the photograph as a token of remembrance. In his influential essay on the effects of the mechanical image upon art, Walter Benjamin notes that it is not coincidental that the first subject of photography was the portrait.[147] Humans originally created art for ritual purposes, so the portrait occupies a "cult value": the photograph becomes an object in the "cult of remembrance."[148] Photographs enable us to venerate our past. They also confirm our mortality through the medium's unknowable and accidental situation, as well as the impossibility of cataloguing reality accurately.[149] Barthes observes that photography cannot be taken to connote or denote anything general or universal because its contingency places it "outside of meaning":[150] photography might come to signify anything other than the particular only "by assuming a mask."[151] This mask is the shifting and mutable meaning and memory that we attribute to the photograph as we appropriate it for our own remembrance purposes. And as we remember through our photographs, we are reminded of our mortality, the strangeness of the passage of time, and the contingency of memory.

Photographs operate as a visual emotional history of our embodiment: through photographs we can observe ourselves getting younger or older, fatter or thinner; our shifting physical abilities; changes in our hair, clothing, or makeup styles; the beginning and ending of relationships; birth and death; and of course, the transformation of our faces and bodies through cosmetic surgery. This history exists at the level of surface, and photography offers assistance for thinking about the body's emotional history as visible on the skin. As the medium of loss and death and as remembrance object, photography possesses an uncanny quality, being simultaneously strange and familiar. The photographic objectification of ourselves (as Barthes puts it, the moment in which we realize that we are shifting positions from being the subject to being the object of the photograph) estranges us from photographs of our past as evidence of aging, just as the effect of gazing into the photographed eyes of someone who is long dead is uncanny. The photograph is a particularly apt site of the double as uncanny because in the double we see everything that we might have become, but did not, the ego-hopes that were demolished due to circumstance, and every action we did not take that maintained our fantasy of free will.[152] This uncanny characteristic of the double is mirrored in the photograph because we not only see our various embodiments at particular points in history but also everything that we might have become. Because of the existence of photographs, we can imagine ourselves as different from how we currently appear. This happens in the past, present, and future: in the photograph's uncanny doubling, not only do we see the possibilities that might have been, but we also see the possibilities that might currently exist and might happen in the future.

These two experiences – the experience of the uncanny double and the experience of looking at a photograph locked in a moment in time that has passed – are a return. Freud holds that repression separates us from an uncanny element or experience.[153] When discussing Jacques Lacan's use

of the term "photo-graphed,"[154] Prosser says this term represents the split
between "reality and representation, between the light and the writing."[155]
The inability of the photograph to reflect back to us the whole moment in
which the photograph was taken parallels the ineptitude and failures of
language. Prosser goes on to explain that Lacan uses the photograph as a
"conductor for the traumatic return of the real,"[156] or the return of the ineffable, incomprehensible trauma that evades reality.[157] In a surface imagination culture that considers cosmetic surgery a viable option to address
the anguish caused by one's body, the prevalence of photographs in our
lives – from family albums to celebrity tabloids – provides a great deal of
material with which to re-envision our appearances in the future or return
to old appearances, all of which is ultimately unsatisfying.

Judith Fryer Davidov confronts the jumbling of time in the experience
of the photograph through John Berger's work: in the photograph, "what
was there" can only be fragmentary, like memory.

> "Before a photograph you search for what was there," John Berger
> writes with wonderful ambiguity about the nexus of memory and
> photography. Memory he understands as a field where different
> times coexist – the time of the subject, of the photographer, of the
> viewer – and as a field that is continuous in terms of the subjec-
> tivity that creates and extends it. "Before" refers not only to con-
> fronting, or standing before, a photograph but also to the fact that
> a photograph implies a time prior to its making and a time after-
> ward, thus linking subject, maker, and viewer. Understanding "what
> was there" can only be fragmentary, like memory, and like photo-
> graphs: before a photograph, the time of its making must literally
> be re-membered.[158]

Photography alters the way we remember, and hence the way we relate
to our bodies. Since a photograph connotes the visual past, present, and
future all at once, a picture of our face or body cannot stand solely as a
representation of a past moment but instead is compared with what has
been, what is, and what will come to be. Barthes describes cameras as
"clocks for seeing,"[159] and photographs offer ephemeral traces of our
bodies, "radiations which ultimately touch me, who am here ... the pho-

tograph of the missing being ... will touch me like the delayed rays of a star. A sort of umbilical cord links the body of the photographed thing to my gaze: light, though impalpable, is here a carnal medium, a skin I share with anyone who has been photographed."[160] The photographic light that we share in photographs envelops our bodily histories and comes to be a skin that envelops time and declares that we were there. This "there" might be a geographical, emotional, familial, temporal, or psychic space that our bodies have inhabited, and in the case of cosmetic surgery the before photograph comes to represent a time of adversity, a time prior to taking control of the situation.

Davis sat in on panels composed of various experts who assessed people's bodies and faces to determine if they were eligible to have their cosmetic surgery covered by the Netherlands' national health care plan. She has reported that in all cases but one she was unable to guess what kind of surgery the individual was seeking.[161] This was also a common thread in my interviews; the participants reported that prior to their surgery, at least one person commented that their bodies or faces were fine the way they were and that they did not need surgery. We do not see our bodies in the same way that we see the bodies of others, in part because we see and think about our bodies photographically. As Barthes remarks, "the Photograph sometimes makes appear what we never see in a real face,"[162] extending Benjamin's earlier comments that the lens can see what the naked eye cannot.[163] This has acute consequences for how we think about our bodies: the photograph is an extrapolation of our own bodies and skins, putting them out on a glossy examining table-album for our scrutiny. Susan Sontag writes ominously about the primary effect of the photograph as a "conver[sion of] the world into a department store or a museum-without-walls in which every subject is depreciated into an article of consumption, promoted into an item for aesthetic appreciation."[164] Because photography can make us consider the body as a consumer item capable of being apprehended for the way it looks and at the same time, in its fixated stillness, reveals to us aspects of ourselves that we might otherwise not see, our history of embodiment is confounded with a peculiar aggregate of stagnation and metamorphosis.

The family album is a productive place to continue to link together the aspects of loss and body history that I have discussed so far in this section. Elizabeth Siegel holds that the family album has two functions: first, it gives us visual and historical material to narrate our identities, strengthening our identity stories; and second, it is a way of amusing others and telling them our stories so they better understand who we are.[165] The makeover's fantasy of "before and after" also permeates the family album because the family album shares the same sense of muddled temporality with makeovers and photography. Lury describes the family album in this way: "The contemporary photographic practices of the family album are making it possible for an individual to discard old selves, to try on personae and compare the multiplicity of subject-effects of retro-ductive self-transformation."[166] Photographs occupy an ambivalent and peculiar place of being a site where we can be posed to appear as we never would in our regular lives, and also where we see others and ourselves reflected most accurately. The mutability of interpretations of our past selves revealed through photographs helps us to construct coherent narratives of our lives that incorporate parallax selves into a singular coherent storyline. Prosser's term "ph/autography" refers to how our authentic engagement with photography is inescapably autobiographical,[167] and the family album demonstrates our powerful autobiographical engagement with photographs. The family album is a site of identity negotiation that parallels the manner in which cosmetic surgery is also fundamentally a negotiation of identity in a surgical culture.

Photography's gaze is evanescent and transformative in relation to identity and appearance in surface imagination practices like cosmetic surgery. Benjamin's essay on photography and film contains a curious passage in which he compares the work of the painter to the work of the magician, and the work of the cameraman (*sic*) to the work of the surgeon. Just as psychoanalysis used surgery as a metaphor to invoke scientific precision, depth, and rigour, so too Benjamin applies the metaphor of surgery to photography. He explains that the painter has a certain respect for the distance between the subject and themselves in their work, and that as a result, the painter's work is a total representation of their subject.[168] Correspondingly, the magician also preserves a certain distance from the sick, only laying hands upon the sick person.[169] The cameraman and the surgeon, on the other hand, view their subjects as fragmented and penetrable, and do not maintain distance between themselves and their subjects, instead reassembling the parts of the person photographed and the patient according to a different law.[170] Benjamin uses this metaphor to illustrate his point that filmic and photographic representations are more relevant to contemporary life than painterly representations because they dig deeply into reality to reveal another hidden aspect.[171]

Benjamin's comparison of surgery and photography illustrates that they share a common configuration of subjectivity and a common surface imagination fantasy. Benjamin is here responding to the surfacing of his culture and the transition toward valuing surface over depth in the construction of identity through surfaces. The conflicting desires for interiority and exteriority, with wholeness and fragmentation, shimmer through this metaphor of photography-as-surgery. Benjamin declares that "the enlargement of a snapshot does not simply render more precise what in any case was visible, though unclear: it reveals entirely new structural formations of the subject."[172] Just as surgery delves into the interior of the body, and as psychoanalysis excavates the unconscious, so too photography presents us with what Benjamin names "unconscious optics."[173] All three discoveries are engrossed with the everyday material that is present but (often) concealed, and all value the surface as signifier. In their convictions that there is a presence that generally goes unnoticed but affects the total person, they are linked through the principle that it is possible for a part of the person to be unknowable (though what each does with this unknowable kernel is quite different). And all three discoveries share a topography of the subject that honours the creation and revealing of an identity that can be observed through the surface.

Photographs invite us to infer, imagine, and fantasize, and this is true especially in surface imagination practices like cosmetic surgery. Photography is an ideal accomplice to cosmetic surgery because the photograph can become a blueprint of what we might like to happen to our faces and bodies through surgery, or an inspiration, or evidence of what has happened. The standards by which we evaluate a face or body as attractive are whether they would photograph well.[174] This is crucial in positioning the camera as essential to cosmetic surgery, because cosmetic surgery prepares the face and body for photography. The photographic eye is "insatiable,"[175] according to Sontag, because it presents us with infinite fragments of the world that are open to interpretation. If we extend this way of looking at the world and the body to the practice of cosmetic surgery, the surface imagination fantasies of cosmetic surgery similarly see the body and face in fragments. Since in a surface imagination culture our bodies can be surgically altered, or to appropriate Sontag's apt phrasing (regarding visual and written representations of individuals), "interpreted"[176] in a variety of ways, the surgical photographic eye is insatiable when it comes to imagining how our bodies and faces might look otherwise.

"Before and After": The History of the Cosmetic Surgery Photograph

The history of photography in cosmetic surgery illustrates the themes of surface imagination and interpretation, which are nowhere more apparent than in the before and after photograph. Blum's astute consideration of the after photograph pulls together several of these threads about photography as a history of embodiment and a loss itself. Photography fuses together science, aesthetics, and business in the history of cosmetic surgery, and by the 1890s the photograph had become an ideal stage on which to demonstrate cosmetic surgery's results, first providing legitimacy and then advertising.[177] This marks a pivotal moment in how *all* bodies began to be conceived as a potential after picture, not just those subject to surgical intervention.

Blum holds that the expansion and popularity of photographic portraits facilitated a metamorphosis in thinking about the body as a "potential after picture of itself."[178] The after representation traces how one's embodiment has altered over time, and at the exact moment that the photograph is taken, it also becomes a before picture. Our photographic selves line up in a sequence of surface imagination images and offer evidence that we have changed (or not changed) according to our desires. When surgeon and patient are making decisions about the potential surgical procedures and desired outcomes, the photograph is the ground upon which both project their anticipation. Undergoing cosmetic surgery means engaging with a procedure whose results will make over the body into a new body that is more suitable for photography, linking the after photo to the "triumph over adversity" story that undergirds surface imagination fantasies about cosmetic surgery.[179] More simply, this photograph offers us hope that one day our fortunes will change, and the photograph comes to hold more legitimacy than the body itself, for two reasons. First, the unruly body of the before photograph has been defeated and is "elegiac in content," to borrow Blum's lovely phrasing.[180] Second, the after photograph stands for an intangible, more attractive afterward for the body, a promise that becomes more important than the body's materiality.

The entanglement of photography and plastic surgery began in the mid-nineteenth century, when plastic surgeon Gurdon Buck brought together the two fledgling technologies to document and provide evidence of his work. He was the first doctor to use before and after photographs to provide substantiation of what cosmetic surgery had achieved.[181] While we now think of this practice as commonplace for many medical procedures, the use of photography in medicine was an innovation, and Buck included photography alongside engravings and casts as verification of surgical results. Significantly, in their historical moment these photographs (and the lithographs based on these photographic images) were the only documents providing an account of Civil War plastic surgery, because the various procedures developed and refined had not yet been described in plastic surgery journals or books.[182] Thus, the very first documents of the development of procedures that form the foundation of contemporary cosmetic surgery practice are photographic and rely on the viewer to read into the visual documents to construct a story about what has occurred. Photographs of before and after transformations are not a contemporary obsession of the cosmetic surgery industry, as we might assume, but rather are the foundation upon which cosmetic surgery has been built. The photograph is central to cosmetic surgery as a document of surface imagination transformations, available for the viewer's interpretations and fantasies.

Figure 2.1 is a photograph taken in 1865 of William Simmons, a Civil War soldier who had surgery to repair the damage done by a shell fragment: both images perform versions of stoic, white masculinity. This valorization of the plastic surgeon through the photograph serves to validate plastic surgery as a procedure that is not undertaken as simple "beauty surgery." I am less interested in the transformations they depict than in how these early before and after photographs establish particular conventions for plastic surgery photography and legitimize the aesthetic surgeon. The soldier wounded by shell fragments and the plastic surgeon who operates on the soldier's face are participants in a serious, nation-building process, positions that authorize surgeries performed in absence of a reason deemed "medically necessary." Thus, the early surgeon was able to develop techniques that would be invaluable to his aesthetic

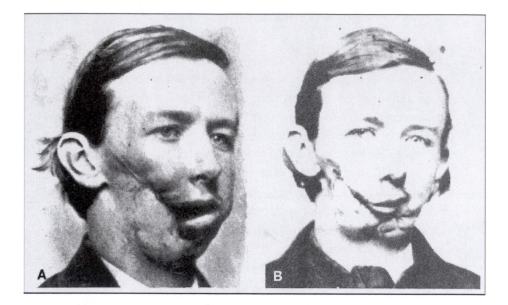

2.1 Gurdon Buck, Case 8, 1865, Wm. Simmons.

surgery practice in a context that was irreproachable. The confluence of photography and the availability of patients to experiment on created a rich opportunity for plastic surgeons interested in surgeries that transformed the appearance of the body. They could document the surface transformations of the body in a way that was simultaneously justifying and promotional. In these early photographic practices, we can see the foreground of contemporary practices in cosmetic surgery photography, such as darkening the before image, manipulating the light to highlight the features that will be operated on, and using eye contact (or lack of eye contact) to communicate the emotional content of the photograph.

The second photograph I wish to consider is from Vilray Papin Blair's article "Underdeveloped Lower Jaw, with Limited Excursion," published in the *Journal of the American Medical Association* in 1909 (Figure 2.2), which follows conventions established since Buck's documentation of plastic surgery in the mid-1800s. This photograph is representative of before and after photographs before the two world wars. The woman is posed in the style of classical portraiture, but the viewer is encouraged to look through a medicalized gaze. The photographs are chronologically positioned in relation to each other in the same way that we read photographs today: left to right, as readers in English would read text. The upper left photograph depicts the face of suffering: with forlorn eyes gazing directly at the viewer, down-turned mouth and droopy eyebrows, the subject confronts us with her sadness. The photograph below is easier to look at, in that it is a side view of the subject, who is no longer looking at us.

In many ways, this photograph is the "objective" evidence of the surgery because it shows us the "underdevelopment" of the chin in relation to the rest of the face. On the right hand side, we see two after photographs that demonstrate what Gilman identifies as a goal of cosmetic surgery: happiness, and thus a better outlook on life. The frontal view of the subject shows a primly dressed woman, with shoulders slightly turned, who gazes into the camera with eyes that demonstrate, according to Blair, that a "happier expression ... is one of the results"[183] of the surgery. As evidence of the psychological benefits of lower jaw surgery, the photograph on the bottom right shows us that her chin has indeed changed. One of the most remarkable strategies evident in this photograph is its use of light and shadow: the photographs on the left use a dark background and shadow (particularly facial shadowing around the eyes and chin) as a means to convey unhappiness and suffering, while the photographs on the right feature a light background that almost absorbs the body of the subject, but uses shadow in a similar way as the before photographs: to emphasize the sinister quality of the feature that has undergone cosmetic surgery.

In the mid-twentieth century, before and after photographs of cosmetic surgery began to change. While we can certainly see some hints of happiness (or at least satisfaction) as an outcome of cosmetic surgery in Blair's before and after photographs, it isn't until the mid-twentieth century that cosmetic surgery photographs are deliberately staged to emphasize happiness. Many emblems of postwar prosperity in North America are structured around surface imagination fantasies, such as the suburban home, the housewife, the domestically made car, or Dior's New Look. These transformations of the appearance of domestic spaces and their inhabitants for public consumption are meant to signify happiness and prosperity, much like the before and after photographs of cosmetic surgery. The shift to prosperity in postwar North America is marked by conflicting and changing ideologies of gender, race, and class, in spite of popular understandings of this time as uniformly restrictive and conformist for women. This can be seen in the popular media of the time which, according to

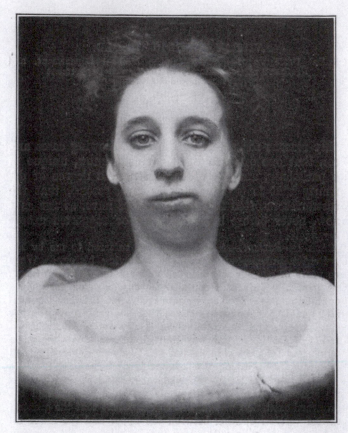

Fig. 1.—Full face of Patient 1 before operation. Notice the lateral position of the chin.

Above and following pages: 2.2a, 2.2b, 2.2c, and 2.2d
Vilray Papin Blair, "Underdeveloped Lower Jaw, with Limited Excursion"

Joanne Meyerowitz, privileged women as homemakers and mothers but presented women engaged in a range of public and private pursuits.[184] However, the caricature of the ideal postwar woman as the white, middle-class housewife and stay-at-home mother is a result of surface imagination fantasies of this period that are held in the contemporary moment. These fantasies are that the rebuilding of the nation after the Second World War can be evidenced in the happy and prosperous bodies of its citizens.

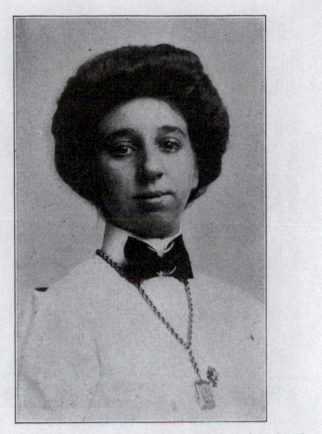

Fig. 3.—Full face of Patient 1 after operation; lateral malposition of chin corrected.

Dr Robert Allen Franklyn's self-promotional memoir, *Beauty Surgeon*, features photographs that are clearly arranged to present a narrative of sadness and despair transformed by cosmetic surgical interventions (in Linda Lee's example, breast implants). The body's surface is the primary site upon which this surgical transformation from loneliness and despair to connection and happiness has occurred, and we see the surgical results through the body's posture, facial expressions, clothing, and the setting of the photographs. As with many before and after photographs from the mid-twentieth century onward, it is actually difficult for the viewer to discern exactly which cosmetic surgery procedures were performed on the

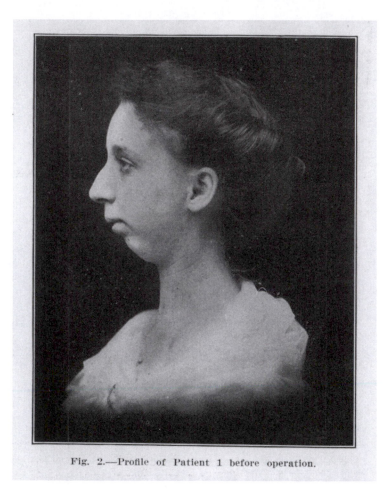

Fig. 2.—Profile of Patient 1 before operation.

patient depicted. As viewers, we are to infer that the physical alteration of the body through cosmetic surgery has altered the emotional and social life of the patient, fulfilling the surface imagination fantasies promised through cosmetic surgery.

The before and after photographs we are accustomed to seeing in magazines and on television are both more and less subtle than their predecessors. Frequently, the subject is positioned underneath fluorescent lighting, without makeup, with hair tied back tightly, and with a drawn or sad expression on her face. The after picture, in contrast, is well lit; makeup is used to enhance the effects of the surgery; her hair has been styled; and she smiles, or at the very least she is shown with an open mouth

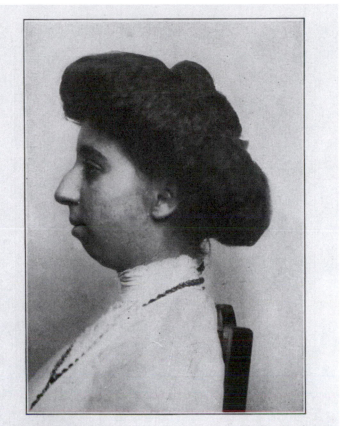

Fig. 4.—Profile of Patient 1 after operation. Notice the change in the relative position of lips resulting from the new position of the body of the lower jaw.

or upturned corners of the mouth. The melodramatic elements of the mid-twentieth century photographs are less present, and the photographs attempt a depiction of cosmetic surgery that holds on to the affective content of the earlier photographs but with a more sanitized and objective feel that positions cosmetic surgery as an inevitable and understandable solution to unhappiness. These photographs combine features of medical evidence of what has happened as a result of the surgery (for advertising purposes) and tabloid-style reporting about the cosmetic surgery of the stars. The photographs demonstrate the unhappiness and suffering of the patient prior to the surgery, and in the after images, all traces of anguish, suffering, or pain that the surgery may have caused must be camouflaged.

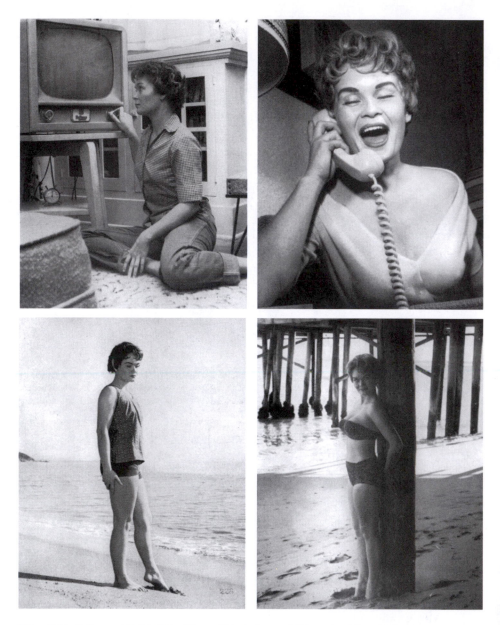

2.3a, 2.3b, 2.3c, and 2.3d "The Story of Linda Lee – A Triumph of Beauty Surgery over Misery"

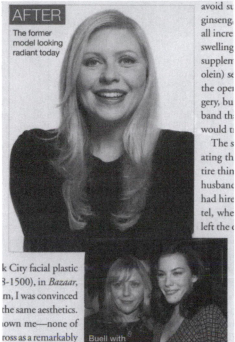

AFTER
The former
model looking
radiant today

avoid su
ginseng,
all incre
swelling
supplem
olein) se
the oper
gery, bu
band th
would t

The s
ating th
tire thin
husband
had hire
tel, whe
left the

k City facial plastic
3-1500), in *Bazaar*,
m, I was convinced
the same aesthetics.
own me—none of
ross as a remarkably

Buell with
daughter
Liv in 2004

about my face, he
facelift, he would BEFORE

2.4 Bebe Buell

The gaze of the photographs no longer belongs to the history of medical photography, but is now situated with the gaze of fashion and advertising photography and makeover culture.

These two photographs come from a popular women's magazine and depict an extraordinary ordinary woman (Figure 2.4, actress Liv Tyler's mother/former model Bebe Buell, from *Harper's Bazaar*) and patient on a cosmetic surgeon's website (Figure 2.5) who had a facelift. Unlike Franklyn's sensational story of Linda Lee, these surgical transformations are more obvious to the viewer, and the emotional content of the photograph is presented with more subtlety. I decided to include them because they are widely available and promise nothing less than total transformation, which is the promise of cosmetic surgery in a surface imagination culture. These photographs are closely linked to the convention of the makeover in highlighting the glamour of cosmetic surgery through the skilful use of cosmetics, hairstyling, and lighting to produce a more dramatic result that can be clearly seen.

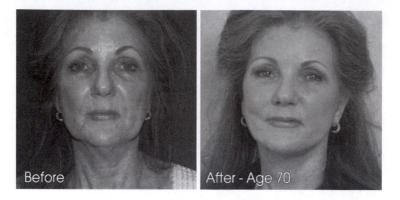

2.5 "Facelift Surgery – Before and After Photo" by Sadi Erfani, MD

However, the alteration of photographs is presently a source of great anxiety and interest in popular culture. Since the photographs we see in magazines are always retouched, they are particularly blamed for women's bad body image and heightened concern about their appearance. The original touch of the button that opened the shutter initiated a loss for the photograph's subject, as she became its image-object, and the re-touch of the photograph by the computer's cursor also severs excess flesh from the body, in a sterile mimesis of cosmetic surgery. These concerns about the authenticity of media images are emphasized by the popular media and downplayed by cosmetic surgeons, and the focus shifts toward a consideration of which cosmetic surgeries are contemptible and which are acceptable.

Conclusion

This chapter offers some background to the circumstances within which my interviewees had their surgeries and the way they narrate their stories.

As a profession, cosmetic surgery continues to struggle for legitimacy, although the current struggle is quite different from the struggle to found the profession over one hundred years ago. Professional medical and surgical organizations have distanced themselves from so-called outlandish cosmetic surgeries by legitimizing their practice on the basis of psychological justifications rather than beauty concerns. Through wartime surgery, cosmetic surgery justified itself on the basis of alleviating psychological suffering and economic disadvantage caused by combat injuries. Since the history of cosmetic surgery grapples with many questions about the relationship between the interior and exterior of our bodies, a strong link exists between the histories of cosmetic surgery and psychoanalysis. The discourse of cosmetic surgery now pervades North American popular culture, assisted by our fantasies of self-transformation. Dissatisfaction with one's life can precipitate the making over of one or more aspects that make one unhappy, and there is a great deal of cultural material that repeats the story of the makeover. Cosmetic surgery has used psychoanalysis and psychology to legitimate its existence and, in its development as a profession, has cultivated a mutually beneficial relationship with the makeover and photography. The historical and contemporary contexts in which cosmetic surgery has developed and continues to develop reveal the parallel stories offered by psychoanalysis and photography, all of which are structured by surface imagination fantasies. As cosmetic surgeons experiment with new techniques that delve deeper than the skin (for example, investigating the role that our muscular structure plays in our appearance), the idea of the interior assumes a different meaning from the psychical. In tandem with the beauty industry, cosmetic surgeons have also successfully created new pathologies out of physiological processes and experiences such as aging and small-breastedness and reconceptualized disfigurement as both a natural and accidental occurrence. To do this, cosmetic surgeons characterized their profession as merciful and in the pursuit of happiness, characterizations that later developed into the surgeon as artist and surgeon as scientist, with their respective interests in universal beauty and scientific pragmatism.

Culturally, cosmetic surgery continues to be troubled by questions about the relationship between our interiority and exteriority, and surface imagination fantasies help cover up that unease. This relationship is not explored by cosmetic surgeons or the popular media, which instead choose to discuss questions about the influence of the media on body image or whether it is morally contemptible that we live in a culture that will assist and encourage women to surgically alter their feet to fit and look good in high heeled sandals or labia to emulate *Playboy* models' vulvas. While these are indeed interesting questions, I think they conceal a much bigger question, one filled with anxiety. *What if it is possible for us to change parts of our lives and emotions through changing the surface of our bodies?* What implications do surface imagination fantasies have for the relationship between our psyches, our bodies, and our culture?

THE PHOTOGRAPH AS REMINDER, EVIDENCE, AND PROMISE

3

"Without the camera, there could be no cosmetic surgery,"[1] Virginia Blum boldly declares. Photography's hold on identity and appearance is evanescent as well as transformative, and photographs are valuable objects for surface imagination practices and technologies like cosmetic surgery. The photograph is the idealized surface of the cosmetic surgery industry, assuming many functions that principally work to distance the patient from the body part to be transformed. It mobilizes the fantasy of a changeable body by providing evidence that change has occurred. It is an object of visual culture that is ultimately other to the self, and the desire to appear attractive in photographs is a result of this otherness. Not only does the photograph serve as a docket of what happened; it offers inspiration for cosmetic surgery through manipulation of its surface and through the multitude of images from which we have to choose when selecting the perfect body part for ourselves. The flattering photograph in particular can be thought of as an idealized skin that presents our body as intact or whole (because it is beautiful), and adequately protected from the exterior world (because it is beautiful).

I had not thought much about the significance of the photograph when I embarked on this project. Indeed, while I planned to outline the function and importance of the before and after photograph within the culture of cosmetic surgery, I did not anticipate that photography would haunt my research in the way that it has. However, this is precisely what the photograph does. A peculiar object, the photograph alienates us from others through its failure to represent a place, time, or person. Many of us are familiar with the experience of showing photographs to another person only to have them flip by the most important one (to us), or we make a disappointed remark such as, "This one really doesn't capture the vastness of this mountain, the way looking at it made me hold my breath." We speak about photography in terms of abduction and killing, as we capture the moment and shoot the picture, apt verbs that point out the deadness inherent within the frozen image. However, the photograph is more akin to the living dead because sometimes there is something within that arrests our gaze and revisits us after the fact. Through the objectification of a moment in time, and as an object in itself, the photograph leads a strange doubled existence. It establishes distance.

A photograph of one's self leads an especially strange life. As I write, I think about a photograph of myself that is in a box on my desk. I am about six or seven years old, wearing a pink, short-sleeved dress with small white flowers, white socks, and red shoes covered with dried mud. My hair is blonde; while I have no recollection of the moment frozen in this photograph, I do recall giving myself a mullet-style cut one evening after returning from the hairdresser's house down the road. My mom had been so pleased that all my hair had reached one length. The sun is on my back, and the front of my body and side of my face are in shadows. Riding a tire swing that runs diagonally and parallel to a large tree branch, I flash a gap-toothed smile at the camera. The bare deciduous trees and muddy corn fields indicate that the photo was likely taken in the spring, and the rural highway runs just below the slanted horizon. I do not remember what it felt like to ride that tire swing, though it looks like fun and I do not appear to be frightened.

This photograph cuts into me. How did I become the adult I am now from this child?[2] I could tell a story about my archaic proclivity toward having fun, the deep split between wanting to please my parents (the wide smile, the tangible pleasure of posing for them) and defy them (the muddy shoes, cutting my finally evened-out hair), or even a narrative that borrows from the fable of the country mouse and the city mouse. I could perform a scholarly analysis of the gendered, raced, and classed locations of this photograph. None of these would answer my question sufficiently because these stories cannot approach the strangeness of our forever-becoming and the terror that over time, the body will do as it pleases in a way that is not at all like the way we can change the details of a photograph.

Cosmetic surgery requires that the patient do just this: take the photograph and examine its minutiae, wonder how the body has changed or why it is the way it is. Steven Connor connects the glossiness of the photographic surface with an idealized skin, an idealization that cosmetic surgery capitalizes on. He argues that the glossy finish remains popular because it invites the touch.[3] The shiny and smooth surface feels good beneath the caress of our fingertips, and we handle glossy photographs with great care. The glossy photograph possesses a "more than human perfection"[4] of a skin, which, according to Connor, occasions both the loving touch and the impulse to tear or cut the photograph in anger or grief. Like our skins, the photograph is vulnerable to time and bears its marks. Connor develops a more hopeful existence of the photographic image than I would. He argues that the image does not necessarily establish distance between its subject and ourselves, but rather that the loving touch we desire to place upon the photographic surface suggests "contiguity between looking and grasping."[5] While I agree that there is a tactile link between the photograph and the skin, I maintain that the distancing effects of the photograph remain paramount, and that this objectifying distance is necessary for cosmetic surgery's existence.

A few participants referred to a particular photograph, or set of photographs, as they illuminated their stories of cosmetic surgery. However, more commonly, the interviewees discussed their bodies *photographically*, or to put it more simply, they used *visual* language that referenced the photograph's promise of transformation. These photographic descriptions surprised me since my interview questions were not written to elicit such commentary. This objective and objectifying language was in sharp contrast to the many emotions the interviewees expressed. While the language of emotions and interiority is a significant and legitimate way to explain one's decision to have cosmetic surgery, my interviews demonstrated that the purportedly objective photographic image is also an important support to cosmetic surgery narratives.

This chapter explores the photograph as the objective and idealized surface of cosmetic surgery. Photography is a medium that connects and distances us from others (and we can say this of the visual realm more generally). However, it also makes our own self an other that we can scrutinize at close range. The photograph is an idealized skin, with its glossy or matte surface, and a metaphorical space that can contain our bodies in a way that we can only dream our skins will.

I divide my consideration of photography and the realm of visual culture into two interrelated themes that emerged from the interview narratives. The first section concerns photography and visual language. I explore the objectification of the body in cosmetic surgery through this discourse, and how this objectification facilitates one's engagement with surgery. In particular, I focus on light as a social phenomenon; discourses of proportion and symmetry; and the split between looking and being looked at as conceptualized through the focal point. I have titled the second section "Snapshots," which refers to the use of actual photographs in narrating cosmetic surgery. In this section, I am concerned with the actual photographs that the interviewees discussed during our conversations. In both sections, I am interested in how the photograph contributes to one's sense of what I am calling an "embodied history" through the concept of surface imagination. What does the photograph accomplish in surgical stories? How does the photograph help the patient fragment and objectify the body in preparation for surgery? When we examine relations of looking in narratives of cosmetic surgery, how might we conceptualize cosmetic surgery in imagistic ways?

The photographic surface operates as an ideal that the patient identifies with, and through this identification the patient self-objectifies and negates the embodied suffering caused by cosmetic surgery in order to more closely identify with the disembodied ideal photograph. The use of the photograph in cosmetic surgery – employing photographic language, in addition to the photograph itself – is an effect or technique of surface imaginations.[6]

Photographic Objectification and Visual Language

When I listened to the interviewees' narratives of cosmetic surgery, I was struck by how the descriptions of their bodies travelled back and forth between establishing a distance from their bodies through the objectivity of photographic language, and drawing closer through referring to their emotional histories of embodiment. The interviewees conceptualized their bodies primarily using the sense of vision, because vision is critical in considering cosmetic surgery as an option to deal with bodily dissatisfaction. Using visual language borrowed from sources as diverse as art history and women's magazines, they distanced themselves from their bodies. This distancing enabled them to consider a physically painful procedure to correct something they perceived as a visible flaw. Considering cosmetic surgery as a route to address grievances with one's body requires the patient to remember, reconstruct, and forget her embodied history. The body's history holds former embodiments that offer proof that the surgeon has done his work to transform the body's surface. Bodies also hold intergenerational histories, including violence and trauma. And yet the patient also has to forget previous bodily traumas and pain in order to agree to have surgery voluntarily and without an authorized medical reason.

The interviewees established this objective distance through objectifying their own bodies using discourse borrowed from the study of art and aesthetics. They employed visual language to understand the benefits of their surgeries in a variety of ways. They described their bodies through relations of looking, which encompassed looking at other bodies, being looked at, and looking at one's self, in addition to applying the aesthetic principles of lighting, proportion, and symmetry to their analyses of their bodies. This visual language smoothed the way for the interviewees' discussions of their body images. In a culture that is paradoxically obsessed with the idealized photographic image (in magazines, for example) and, at the same time, with the detrimental effects of the idealized photograph on body image, talking about the body image in relation to one's cosmetic surgery is practically a requirement for these narratives. In the following chapter, I elaborate on how the skin contributes to one's sense of body image, and I note here that my definition of body image fits more closely with the work of psychoanalyst Paul Schilder. This is because Schilder takes body image more seriously from the perspective of the individual experience than does a feminist analysis of body image, which holds that the individual experience is mistaken or the result of false consciousness.[7] However, the interviewees frequently discussed body image through a feminist-informed lens, and so they undermined their own body images as unimportant because they were not "real." These connected themes demonstrate that, for many of the interviewees, the photograph is a critical surface imagination support in establishing a body image.

Presence or absence of light enables or hinders our ability to look. Light is an elusive and essential quality in art, used to emphasize and conceal features in the subject of an artwork in techniques like chiaroscuro, and even as a medium in light art. The quality of a light can make a setting appear stark and cold (fluorescent lighting in a hardware store, for example) or warm and soft (the light of the setting sun). A light can either cast shadows on the body that obscure features we want to hide, or it can emphasize these features to make them more grotesque than in our worst nightmares.

One of the questions I asked interviewees was, "What memories and emotions do you associate with this part of the body?" Most discussed particular incidents that brought to mind the shame, discomfort, or sadness they felt about those parts of their bodies, but Tigerlily's response was different. I distributed the interview questions by email prior to the interviews so that the interviewees would know in advance what I was interested in discussing, and in order to encourage a more thoughtful response. Tigerlily indicated prior to our meeting that she did not understand this question and did not think she had anything to contribute regarding the subject. I offered some clarification through my emails, reminded her that she could choose to answer or not answer any question, and at the time of our interview, I asked the question to see if she had thought of anything since she had last emailed me. She began her response in a tentative way, as though searching for some memory of her face that she could share with me, and that would be useful for my project. Then she told me that she lives in three homes throughout the year, depending on the season. She explained that the light in each home is quite different, and that she prefers the light in her home in the Caribbean because "it's just the way the window is in relation to the sun and maybe the colouring in the room," which make her "feel good in the morning." She continued, "Your own reflection works back into how you feel about yourself, and how you present yourself to the world ... but it's strange when you think of the lighting factor. And I'm talking more about daylight, the addition of artificial light doesn't seem to make that much difference, it's the, like, when you look in the morning, in the light, in the early afternoon." Tigerlily evocatively conveys the importance of light to how she perceives her face, and describes what kinds of light make her feel good (the ideal light in the Caribbean) and bad (the unflattering light in Canada). Artificial light does not matter to Tigerlily's perception of how she looks; it is rather the natural sunlight that affects her mood. And so it is not surprising that Tigerlily was in one of her Canadian homes when she decided to have a face and eye lift. Tigerlily's narrative presumes that cosmetic surgery enables her to feel the same way about her face in Canada as she does in the Caribbean.

Tonya also references light during our interview discussion. For Tonya, though, the abundance or lack of light connotes exposure and concealment. Since she was embarrassed about her large breasts, Tonya said that she never went topless in front of other people until her appointment with her surgeon. At her consultation appointment, it was "very odd … to have someone so casually manhandling you … with the lights on" "when [your breasts are] such a heavy source of shame." When I asked her how her relationship with her body changed after her surgery, Tonya replied that she felt "way more comfortable to have sex with, like, with lights[, a]s opposed to in pitch black." In contrast to Tigerlily, who viewed light as having a flattering or unflattering effect on the overall appearance of her face, for Tonya the darkness operated as a secure cloak, and the light left her feeling uncomfortably exposed.

While these stories diverge, both demonstrate what Mikkel Billie and Tim Flohr Sørenson call the sociality of light. While a more conventional analysis of light might focus on its materiality, or light as a metaphor for moral superiority, the sociality of light suggests that light exists as a part of social life that is culturally specific.[8] Thus, light is not only shed on our environments but creates them; reflects our identities, cultural backgrounds, and morality; and can expose or conceal features of our social life. Tigerlily's narrative expresses the emotional qualities of light that depend on geographical location. In the northern hemisphere, many people cope with a lack of energy and depression due to seasonal affective disorders (SADs), which are primarily the result of the quantity and quality of daylight during the northern winter. I am not suggesting that Tigerlily herself is expressing symptoms of SADs; however, she is conveying an affective quality of light that causes her to regard her face in a critical and negative manner. Tonya, on the other hand, discusses light in terms of revealing and disguising, and tries to avoid the intimate glare of the light.

Tonya's refusal to allow fully lit access to her body might be considered a response resulting from the dominant visual culture's strategies of illuminating the idealized body to highlight its beauty and camouflaging the de-idealized body to hide its defects. This is a social relation of light that is culturally specific to surface imagination-oriented cultures. For example, in a cultural context that privileged touch, Tonya might be more inclined to deny physical, rather than visual contact with her breasts; in such a context she might not experience any discomfort about the size of her breasts. In a visually dominated surface imagination culture, however, the impressions that can be obtained from the surface are taken to be representative of the self.

Proportion and Symmetry

Another lesson from art history present in the interviews is the importance of proportion and symmetry. The demand for balance in the discourse of aesthetics has been a critical support for many surgical procedures for as long as modern cosmetic surgery has existed. A commonly held belief is that humans evolutionarily prefer symmetry of the face and body and proportionate bodies (leading to the view that, for example, a 0.7 waist to hip ratio is a universal ideal for women's bodies). The appeal to proportion and symmetry fuses together the surgeon-artist and surgeon-scientist, since it weds beauty and measurement.

I asked Leah to describe her reasons for seeking out cosmetic surgery on her breasts, and she gave me a very detailed account based on her body's disproportion.

THEY Never Really Did Anything for Me (Leah, breast reduction and lift)

I'm looking in the mirror.
Body image-wise I was never really thrilled, everything started really big on top.
Then you get to my stomach,
Small legs,
Like an upside-down pear.
The way my body was proportioned,

THEY

just never really did anything for me.

Like I was noticeably bigger on top,
I was never really thrilled,
and it was something I was self-conscious about when I was younger.
The way my body was proportioned, I was never really thrilled.

Leah's account of her body's proportions explains her decision to seek surgery in the terms that the surgeon might also employ to justify it, whether as a surgeon-artist or a surgeon-scientist. This is particularly so in Leah's case, where the doctor would have had to justify the surgery to a provincial health insurance board in order to obtain coverage. Through recourse to a scientifically articulated aesthetics based on a combination of classical aesthetics and sociobiology, Leah's body is shown to be out of proportion. However, this is only half of the account Leah gives of her proportions. The other half borrows from women's magazines, which suggest that all faces and bodies can be categorized as one type or another, and that knowledge of your type can help you select the correct cosmetics, hairstyle, and clothing. Women's faces are divided into shapes (oval, square, rectangle, circle, heart, triangle), and bodies are divided into fruits (apple, pear, banana). Leah's description of her body as shaped like "an upside-down pear" demonstrates probable knowledge of these systems of classification, and she alternates this framework with a medical aesthetics.

Diana, who had just four pounds of fat removed from her body, explained to me that one of her reasons for wanting liposuction was that the fat was not equally distributed. When describing her first appointment with her surgeon, she said,

[The surgeon's nurse] looked at my stomach and my love handles, and this is out of order but um, I was also really asymmetrical, like there was a lot more fat on the one side of the love handles than the other and that also bothered me. But she looked at that, and there was ... definitely was enough fat there and she said, you know, like we can take care of that, we can take it right down basically to like where you want it to be. And then I asked her about my thighs and she looked at my thighs and she said, we wouldn't do them, because there's, like there's not, there's not really a problem and there's a chance that they would end up lumpy so we wouldn't like, do that.

For Diana, this confirmation of her asymmetry is especially important. Diana is recovering from an eating disorder, and she presented herself to me as someone who was hyper-aware of the possibility for an unrealistic assessment of her body. Throughout the interview she oscillated between presenting her interest in her love handles and abdomen as (in her words) "neurotic" and as justified. She acknowledged that while she might not have the most objective outlook on her body, she nevertheless wanted liposuction and felt that it would alleviate some of the negative feelings she had about her body. Symmetry is a device that connects Diana's assessment of her body with another person's (the surgeon's nurse) and justifies some of Diana's concerns about her fat distribution as neutral observations. While the nurse and surgeon informed Diana that she would not turn out "perfect" (by which they meant perfectly symmetrical), Diana's surgery promised to at least make her more symmetrical. Here symmetry is an objective qualifier. In contrast, when Diana told the surgeon's nurse that she wanted to have liposuction on her thighs, the nurse responded that because there was nothing wrong with her thighs it would be impossible to obtain surgery on them. It is interesting that Diana presented this event as a test and affirmation of the quality of the surgeon and her screening process, even though Diana was genuinely asking for liposuction for her thighs. In this way, Diana's decision to have liposuction on her back was corroborated by the surgeon's nurse through the standard of symmetry, and surgery on her thighs was dismissed as unnecessary – a "neurotic" worry, as Diana characterizes it.

Looking and Being Looked At

The criteria discussed above possess conspicuous neutrality because of their references to aesthetic categories such as light, proportion, and symmetry. While these experiences of looking at the body happen in relation to the world, the interviewees also individually assess them. In contrast, the interviewees also talked about their visual experiences of their bodies by directly addressing the complicated pact between looking and being looked at. While the former assume an implicit looker, the latter focus more directly on the conditions of being looked at.

John Berger reflects on looking and being looked at in his classic book *Ways of Seeing* (1972), a discussion of the representation of women throughout art history. Berger's critique focuses on the subjective elements of looking (at art), and he argues that the contemporary visible world is centred on the looker. The present model of perspective in the history of Western painting positions the viewer as the omnipotent centre of the visible world. The effect of this model is that vision is conceptualized as non-reciprocal.[9] Berger argues – on the basis of a curious confluence of psychoanalytic and Foucauldian theory that has been rehearsed countless times by other theorists since – that in the Western world, to be a woman means to be an image. Women must watch themselves (becoming the surveyed), and are "continually accompanied by an image of [themselves]."[10] Women's interior surveyors are gendered as masculine and women turn themselves into objects (specifically objects of vision). Forty years later, it is considered more productive to think of modes of vision as occupying masculine and feminine *positions of power* (rather than biologically determined roles); however, Berger's argument is significantly more complicated than the common understanding of objectification, circulating in popular media, as something that happens unilaterally to women by men. Further, it anticipates the prevalence of surface imaginings of the body through photography found in contemporary North American cultures.

Leah said that when she looked at her body immediately following surgery, she noticed that her breasts were no longer the "focal point." Prior to her breast reduction, Leah thought of her breasts as the first thing that others' eyes were drawn to. In particular, Leah was concerned about other people staring at her stretch marks. Thus, Leah described her breasts in exactly the same way that the focal point in art is defined: as a point where lines of sight converge or diverge, in the same way that our eyes are drawn to the vanishing point in perspectival painting. What Leah appreciated about her body after the surgery was that it was made visually whole since there was no longer a particular point (stretch marks or breasts) that others stared at before looking at the rest of her body. Leah presented the narrative of her breasts before surgery in terms of how she appeared to others. Interestingly, she also said that after surgery she did not want others to notice that her breasts were smaller, suggesting that Leah wanted her breasts to blend in with the rest of her body so that she no longer had to deal with the attention of others upon her breasts.

Tonya and Melinda, the other interviewees who had breast surgeries, shared similar stories about breasts as a focal point of looking. Tonya stated that she hoped her breast reduction surgery would take away the attention she received because of her breasts:

> You know, and I knew exactly how much space I sort of took up because of my boobs, and I didn't like it, like I just wanted to be more, fly on the wall, more anonymous, less noticed and all that kind of stuff, because you get noticed when you have big, like big boobs like people check you out and whatever ... Even though, it was oftentimes in a positive way I still felt like, you know, pain.

Her breasts prohibited her from occupying public space in an unexceptional way, and the attention she received, while often positive, was not welcomed because it was based on a non-reciprocal look. Melinda wanted her breasts augmented because she appreciated the way they looked when she was nursing and pregnant; however, she had concerns about breast augmentation:

> And I actually got them done but they're just like, similar to when I was nursing, small, and natural, they're similar, I didn't want it to look you know, huge or unnatural but I just, you know, it's not like I wanted everybody to be looking at me, like looking at my boobs or anything, it was more of a private thing for me.

While Melinda did not complain about having breasts that are noticed because of their size, she emphasized that wanting more attention was not one of the reasons she sought breast augmentation.

Leah, Tonya, and Melinda each resisted being looked at in a sexualized manner that fetishized their breasts into fragmentary pieces of their bodies. Their motivations for breast surgeries focused on considering their bodies as an entirety through making the breasts disappear in one way or another. While Tonya and Melinda both described experiencing great pleasure through their breasts, they wanted that pleasure to be private and not exhibitionistic (Leah, on the other hand, did not describe pleasure originating from her breasts at all). Here, looking at the breasts is an amalgamation of a mode of looking that privileges the seer (who possesses the power to determine what is looked at) and the logic of the photograph (which fragments the body as a scene that can be broken into its component pieces and restructured). The problems that Tonya and Leah experienced because of their large breasts, and the problem that Melinda anticipated, originated not in their own perceptions of their bodies, but in how others perceived their bodies. They did not challenge what they saw when they looked at their own bodies, or what they thought others were looking at when regarding their bodies. The visual apprehension of their breasts was considered inevitable, even if unjust.

Diana's narrative, on the contrary, presented her internalized look as significantly less objective than Leah, Tonya, and Melinda's narratives, and she stated that the way she looks at her body is not the same as the way others perceive her body. She presented her concerns about the fat she had removed as "obsessions," suggesting an irrational fixation, and relied on the objective gaze of the nurse to determine what parts of her body did or did not require liposuction. Diana also stated that she keeps a very different standard for her own body than she does for others. While she associated the fat that was removed with not being fit, she also said that she does not have "associations of … laziness with … overweightness" (as a common stereotype), and that she would "absolutely never look at someone who's overweight and think they, they should feel that way." Diana was very knowledgeable about the discourse of eating disorder recovery, and as a result treated her own evaluation of her body as suspect. She talked about her body in a way that emphasized the subjective characteristics of looking and the impossibility of seeing one's own body as others see it. Diana privileged her own perception of her body in spite of its subjectivity, and was more concerned with addressing her "obsessions" than accepting the perceptions of others as valid.

After she had liposuction, Diana was unable to look at her body.

I was like really nervous to look at my own body when I first woke up like, the nurse came in and [she] had to like [change] bandages or whatever and she changed them and like, and I was kind of looking at the nurse and she, she told me that I could look, and I was like, this is weird, like I felt like I needed permission to look at my own body, actually I was just really nervous about it.

This nervousness stood in contrast to Diana's concern prior to her surgery with how the liposuction would look (rather than being concerned with the possibility for adverse side effects, for example), and instead had to do with her body image. She continues:

I think ... for me the most interesting thing about it was ... if ... psychoanalysts say that ... your image of your body is, like your ego is largely an image of your body, and then, so I knew there was going to be, like I kind of, I just kind of didn't look really closely, and that night, that night I was supposed to, you go home, and I was supposed to change the bandage and I did, but I didn't kind of do it in front of a mirror, like I kind of still was really nervous about looking at it, and then, it got swollen and I was still really nervous about looking at it, and I would, I would kind of like, you wear this, this thing that um, like it's kind of a stiff thing that, holds everything in place, I guess ... and so, I kind of didn't really like to take that off, I kind of just wanted it all to heal before I looked at it. And I think that, like, if you have an image of, like if you've had an image of your body, and *I kind of had an absence of an image of my body* because I didn't, because I was nervous to look at it, and also, it was going to get, it was getting swollen soon after, so I didn't really know what it would look like. So I had this absence of an image of my body ... which I found really strange [my emphasis].

In this lengthy passage, Diana is working through several concerns that originate from her firm adherence to her particular conceptualization of her body, which is a purely surface imagination understanding. After the surgery she was worried about what the changes in her body would turn out to be, and also what they would mean. While all participants shared similar concerns in terms of what their changed body meant to them, Diana was especially concerned because she had not previously established an objective foundation upon which to base her judgment. This is not to say that Diana does not also resort to professional justification of her complaint; it is clear from this excerpt that Diana explains her subjectivity through her understanding of the psychoanalytic concept of the bodily ego. To have an absence of an image of her body is strange to Diana, but we can imagine that it would also signal a time of respite. Due to the insistence on her subjective evaluation of her own body, Diana attempts to manage the unpredictability of the surgical outcome by resisting the formation of a new visual incarceration until the traumatic healing process has finished. Immediately following her recovery period, Diana was quite pleased with her outcome; however, even though we spoke less than three months after her surgery, she was already beginning to feel dissatisfied with her body again. These "body image issues," as Diana classifies them, can be thought of as a constellation of images of her body that Diana carries and that are related to the way that she visually perceives her body. Diana's story in particular captures the difficulties of negotiating identity through images and the infinite demands expressed in images.

Since Diana didn't want to look at her body after her surgery, her story might be characterized as *not looking enough* at the body because of the intense intimacy between her body and mind: looking at the body would also be taking a chance that the surgery had not had its desired effect. Contrarily, Tonya's story could be thought of as *too much looking* that led to a depersonalization of her body. A key concept in this interview is Tonya's *non-ownership* of her breasts, which is linked specifically to the appearance of her breasts and the practice of looking. She introduced this concept when she described going to the "boob specialist" who demonstrated the breast reduction procedure by "folding them under" and manipulating them "like they weren't [hers]." She thought that it was very "odd" for the surgeon to be looking at her breasts because they were "a heavy source of shame," and this shame was evoked when the surgeon looked at her breasts in full light. The doctor took front and side photographs to send to a provincial review panel (a "faceless panel of doctors" who are nonetheless quite capable of looking) that would determine whether Tonya was eligible for provincial health insurance coverage (proving that the reasons were medical, not aesthetic), another factor contributing to Tonya's feelings of not possessing her breasts. These feelings of estrangement from her breasts appear as a defence against the highly invasive nature of the consultation and subsequent surgery.

After the surgery, Tonya's feelings of non-ownership were particularly pronounced. She said that her surgical breasts were "not in any way [hers]." She compared her situation to that of an amputee in a novel and what she erroneously calls "false memory syndrome."[11] Tonya compared the itch of a ghost limb (amputated leg) with her chest: she said, "[I] felt like they had removed my entire chest and put on someone else's breasts." She imagined that if someone had attached a new arm, she would feel like that arm was not her own arm and would not really care about the fate of the new arm. Tonya described this strange phenomenon as "kind of amazing," and she correlated this feeling to her breasts. All of her anxiety and shame focused on her breasts vanished, since she did not experience her breasts as belonging to her. Even though she felt like her breasts were "scarred," "disgusting," and "ugly," and she had to do things she found difficult, like being topless with her mother as she applied crème to the scars, she felt fine because she did not perceive her breasts as her own. This feeling remained for a long time, making the possibility of brushing her breasts up against someone else no longer a worry because they felt like "phantom breast[s]."

It took Tonya years before her reconstructed breasts felt "like a sexual object that is my object," as opposed to a "belly button" (her choice of a non-sexual body part). She likened her story of reconfiguring her body image with a smaller-breasted body to the story of a former pregnant classmate who described feeling like "she couldn't squish between two people when she was walking down a hallway or something, and she was always used to knowing exactly how big her body was." Tonya identified strongly with the feeling of not being sure of her spatial surroundings after her body was changed through surgery. She felt okay about wearing tight clothing since her breasts did not feel as though they belonged to her, and her scars did not bother her as much as she expected for this very reason. Tonya was quite invested in maintaining the power to control visual access to her breasts. A housemate at the time asked her a lot of questions about her surgery, including whether the surgeon had changed the size of her nipple and what it looked like. Tonya answered his questions honestly and felt "very happy" about answering in an open and confident manner, and even offered to show him her breasts. His response, however, was to say, "Oh god, no!" and he later said that it was gross and he did not want to see her scars. Tonya was "kind of hurt and pissed off" and wanted to say, "Fuck you buddy … these breasts … are … great … and you don't even want to see them?" She imagines that he thinks "very clearly, oh god no I don't want to see your disgusting breasts, they have like scars on them!" It appears that what Tonya wanted was not necessarily a bar on visual contact with her breasts by others. She said that it troubled her that the breast reduction accomplished the desired effect of diverting the stranger's gaze but also diverted the wanted gaze of her housemate. The unwilling housemate and the too-willing stranger each eschew Tonya as gatekeeper in their particular ways, and part of what Tonya accomplishes through the non-ownership of her post-surgical breasts is a minimizing of this impact on her post-surgical self. Tonya's story captures the desire to control the body in surface imagination fantasies, including controlling the reception of one's body by others.

Leah and Tigerlily also presented their surgeries as means to address body image, though in a less pronounced manner than Tonya and Diana. Due to her dissatisfaction with the disproportion of her body, Leah said, "body image-wise [she] was never really thrilled." She did not reflect much on her body image throughout her narrative, and in fact resisted making her story entirely about fixing a bad body image. Leah indicated that she has always been a pretty confident person, and through her confidence was able to fend off some of the potentially more devastating effects of being unhappy with her appearance. Nevertheless, Leah did present her discontent with her breasts as "definitely a bit of a body image issue in one sense," and positioned the stretch marks as the flip side of the coin (a "self-conscious issue" in her words). As with much of her interview narrative, Tigerlily presented the relationship between body image and her surgery in a pragmatic fashion. She stated simply, "[Y]our own reflection works back into how you feel about yourself, and how you present yourself to the world." This statement was made in tandem with her discussion of the importance of lighting for her perception of her face, and she did not elaborate on it. But it summarizes perfectly the surface imagination fantasy of the deep connection between interior and exterior that is projected outward through the surface of the body.

Speculations on Visuality and the Bodily Ego

The portions of the interview narratives that were the most troubling and difficult for me to witness were concerned with the self-objectification of the body into a surface. They highlighted just how imperfect a solution cosmetic surgery is in addressing the difficulties of inhabiting a body in a cultural context that demands constant attention to improving the body's surface, a contemporary demand that conflicts with desires for stability in identity and embodiment. The women I spoke to were very happy with the results of their surgeries, and yet they tempered their enthusiasm with embodied complaints of numbness, pain, imperfect results, or post-surgical complications. Many also had to negotiate less than perfect relationships with their surgeons, and needed to figure out a way to deal with this asymmetrical power relationship. And all these conditions were tolerated for voluntary surgeries with potentially lethal risks in order to change the appearance of a part of their bodies.[12] Clearly something very serious is at stake here for the interviewees. What psychic distress does cosmetic surgery promise to alleviate for those who undergo it, and what relationship does this function have with the visual objectification of one's own body?

These concerns dovetail with Kaja Silverman's project in *The Threshold of the Visual World*, particularly with her critique of vision's dominance in establishing identifications and idealizations. She is also interested in the limits of vision and the normative power of the gaze. Beginning with Silverman's elaboration of the distinction between the proprioceptive and exteroceptive egos, I extend this discussion into a consideration of the idealization of images and visual language in the interview narratives.

Silverman begins her analysis of visuality with Freud's bodily ego, a concept that apparently resists the separation between the psychical and the biological. However, Freud's bodily ego was not just a cutaneous entity: Freud converted the bodily ego into a visual image. Freud's writing is permeated with visual imagery and metaphor (one of the reasons I find his work so compelling), something that Lacan later took up as problematic. In his mirror stage essay and in *Seminar I*, Lacan emphasizes that the specular image of one's own ego has an inclusionary and exclusionary role vis-à-vis other images; that is to say, our self-image delimits what images are acceptable and unacceptable to our own ego.[13] Silverman states that by Lacan's *Seminar VII*, this ego image becomes the "limit" of the "self-same body," a limit that challenges the postmodern ideal of endless identificatory possibilities.[14] The "self-same body" regulates the images that we can accept and see, suggesting that the bodies we can love are limited by our ego's image of our own body, as well as culturally normative images. Silverman shifts from this understanding of the bodily ego, using James Strachey's footnotes to "The Ego and the Id," to the view that as the visual imago permits the ego to think of the body as a separate object, we come to think about the body as belonging to us through tactile sensations of the skin.[15] In my discussions of skin as the de-idealized surface of cosmetic surgery in the following chapter, I discuss further what it means to situate identity at the level of the skin's surface from the position of Freud's bodily ego.

Schilder's postural model of the body in *The Image and Appearance of the Human Body* (1935) emphasizes the role of touch in the formation of the ego. Schilder suggests that our bodily egos are being meticulously constructed and taken apart all the time, and that cutaneous sensations play a critical role in this creation and destruction. The exterior world comes to our bodily ego through touch, which can be thought of as "social influence." Silverman argues that in Schilder, the "desires addressed to the body" form a sense of the "outline of the skin."[16] Schilder's postural model of the body, while also invested in the importance of the visual imago in ego formation and body image, brings back Freud's insights about touch and the bodily ego. He claims that the visual and the sensational aspects of the ego are in essence unified, because they are integrated with one another through the integration of the two senses.[17] Silverman introduces another figure in the history of psychoanalysis, Henri Wallon, to give an account of the bodily ego that does not consider the sensational ego and the visual imago to be so closely psychically connected.[18] The concepts of the exteroceptive and proprioceptive egos – which I find very useful in analysing the interview narratives – emerge here.

In Wallon's theory, the unification of the exteroceptive ego (or the visual imago) and the proprioceptive ego (or the sensational ego) is difficult and always fragile due to their competing structures and aims. The Lacanian baby jubilantly and instantaneously mis-recognizes herself in the mirror as whole and self-sufficient, and psychically incorporates this imaginary and complete image.[19] This incorporation, as Silverman notes, takes much longer in Wallon's description of the baby's relation to her mirror image. Wallon's baby goes through a series of relationships to her mirror image, extending from an initial love relationship with the image, considering the image as a double or rival, bewilderment that the image is flat and cold rather than warm like skin, making contact with the mirror in various ways (hitting or licking) while considering the image an ally, and gesturing or looking at the mirror image when the baby is called to or mentioned.[20] Silverman notes that whereas the Lacanian baby instantaneously assimilates the imaginary image, the Wallonian baby spends a great deal of time considering the image as separate from herself (from twenty weeks to fifteen months). Silverman calls this "identity-at-a-distance,"[21] a process by which the baby has the opportunity to think of herself as other through the mirror image, rather than as identical to the mirror image.

The second related aspect of Wallon's theory that Silverman distinguishes from Lacanian psychoanalysis is that the Lacanian baby needs only the mirror image in order to distinguish a psychical sense of "self." In contrast, the Wallonian baby has more work to accomplish, for she must bring together this mirror image (exteroceptive ego) with her sense of what is interior and exterior to her body (the domain of the proprioceptive ego). Thus, we can think of proprioceptivity as the sense that we have of our bodies as our own. The proprioceptive ego in Wallon is formed of the cutaneous and muscular sensations of the body, or in other words, the constellation of sensory experiences that accumulate in the body and are perceived as having interior or exterior origins: significantly, this is a non-visual way of conceptualizing psychic subjectivity and development.[22] What is most useful about Wallon's theories of exteroceptivity and proprioceptivity is that there is no assumption that the visual image has any relationship whatsoever to our sensational perceptions of our bodies.

The tenuous connection between our proprioceptive and exteroceptive egos is an important one for thinking about cosmetic surgery, not to mention the social categories of gender and race more generally. Cosmetic surgery can be conceptualized as a technique through which an individual attempts to bring together these disparate images and sensations of themselves in a cultural milieu that privileges the surface. In different ways,

each interviewee discussed feeling that her body somehow did not appear
the way it ought to. The consistent emphasis on the image in the mirror
(or photograph), the imagined image that others would take in, and visual
descriptors of the body indicate that the visual image or proprioceptive
ego troubled the interviewees in some way or another. Wallon's theory
does not pathologize the feeling that something is amiss with the image
that we confront in the mirror and through the eyes of others, but instead
thinks about how the mirror image enables us to "other" ourselves in a
manner that is essential to cosmetic surgery. However, I would add that
this othering cannot be as profound in the mirror image as it is in the photographic image, which is the image of surface imagination *par excellence*.
This is because the mirror image is instantaneous, fleeting, and provides
us with a glimpse of ourselves in the present. It is much fleshier than the
photographic image, and we can make our mirror image react to our presence, just as the Wallonian baby licks and touches the mirror image. The
mirror image is certainly employed in cosmetic surgery fantasies and plans,
but its lifelike quality makes it less useful than the photographic image for
the objectification of the skin's surface that is necessary to imagine
cosmetic surgery. Through the union (even if it might be only attempted,
or even if it is only partially successful) of the proprioceptive and the exteroceptive ego, the mirror image becomes an othering image that belongs
to us. The photographic image, on the other hand, belongs to no one
and everyone, and exists as an othering image that facilitates a more
self-objectifying gaze through surface imagination. Significantly, through
the photograph we are able to share our self-objectifying gaze with others
and invite them to participate in the surface imagination fantasies of our
bodies latent in the photographic surface.

Snapshots

Without the physical photograph, the cosmetic surgery industry would
have very little to shore up its practices and promises. The photograph
offers critical support to the narratives of how the procedure will unfold
and how it happened. The functions of photography in cosmetic surgery
were emphasized in the interview narratives, particularly two frequently
overlapping modes of photography: medical evidence and before and

after photographs. Medical evidence photographs are taken by medical professionals to augment their portfolio, display on their website, or send off to insurance boards to secure coverage for various procedures. These photographs are used largely for economic and advertising reasons. Photographs that provide medical evidence are often, but not necessarily, organized in the before and after sequence discussed in the previous chapter. Before and after photographs can be taken not only by medical professionals but also by the patient or other photographers (for example, in magazines). These photographs offer reassurance or confirmation that cosmetic surgery indeed *does* something to the body or face, hopefully by way of improvement. While the medical evidence mode of photography incorporates the elements of before and after, it takes an extra step to differentiate itself from non-medical photography. The use of photography by a cosmetic surgeon is symbolically weighted through the connections between official state and medical photography, a strategy that better secures patient trust. Magazine photography is a method through which bodies that do not exist in reality come to be idealized, and can be thought of further as cosmetic surgery's non-replicative ideal.

Evidence

Photographs that count as medical evidence share a lineage with other evidentiary state photographs of persons, such as police photographs of crime scenes and mug shots, driver's licenses, immigration certificates and passports, military records, and scientific trials. These photographs are not imbued with the affective charge of the family snapshot, but they are given a special status. Instead of serving as an object that aids our memories of past events, persons, and places, the state photograph is an object that offers evidence to representatives of the state and verifies our identity to these official others. The way we pose our faces and bodies is prescribed by the representative of the state who photographs us, though very rarely do they need to instruct us on the state photograph's conventions. Usually these photographs are frontal face shots, but we also hold our bodies rigid and upright during the photographing. We may be allowed to smile slightly, as in driver's licenses, but often it is verboten to smile into a state photograph. Most of the state photographs that non-state representatives have access to are quite small (around 3 cm x 3 cm). These characteristics of the state photograph bestow on it a certain objectivity, and do not invite questions about whether or not that photograph has been altered.[23]

The Lights On, No Less! (Tonya, breast reduction and lift)
I don't think anybody had ever seen my breasts with the lights on before.
She had to take some pictures of me.
With the lights on, no less!

Those pictures then get sent to some kind of
... review panel ...
to see whether or not it would actually be covered.
I don't know who the panel is made up of.
In my memory, it was like,
faceless panel of doctors.

They look at the notes and the photos,
and they say
– YES, it's a medical necessity, or
– NO, it's not a medical necessity.
They get to decide whether or not it's covered surgery.

Aside from this fifteen minute meeting that I had with this one specialist,
This review committee then basically is looking at your breasts and saying,
"Yeah, they're too big."
"Yeah, they're too ugly."
"Yeah, they're too saggy."
"Sure, we'll pay for your surgery because you don't fit into this idea of what women's breasts should look like."

People are like waiting for like kidney operations,
but, "If you want to be a more like, conventionally attractive woman, we'll help you do that really fast."

When a cosmetic surgeon decides to photograph the patient, he or she is consciously or unconsciously borrowing from the authority of the state photograph. Taking photographs legitimates the procedure, and indicates to the patient that despite cosmetic surgery's reputation for vanity and frivolity, she is about to undergo a serious medical procedure that requires commensurate evidence. The fact that the patient often never views these images further saturates them with an official evidentiary quality due to this restricted access. Because Tonya's breast reduction was performed in Ontario, she was eligible to have her surgery covered by the Ontario Health Insurance Plan (OHIP). Both Tonya's and Leah's narratives confirmed my previous understanding of the reasons many people give for breast reduction surgeries in Ontario:[24] the appearance of large breasts and difficulty fitting into clothing is significantly more troublesome than back pain and related reasons used to qualify for insurance coverage. Both Tonya and Leah discussed lying to their surgeons about the amount of pain they experienced. And Tonya even got caught in her lie by the "boob specialist," who asked her for specifics about her back pain that Tonya was unable to satisfactorily provide. Tonya's appointment with the "boob specialist" who secured the insurance coverage further contradicted this unspoken pact to avoid discussing the appearance of the breasts and focus instead on pain, because this specialist took photographs as a part of the consultation appointment. Why would a specialist take photographs of Tonya's breasts if the surgery's purpose was primarily to alleviate pain? Why wouldn't the specialist try to rule out other potential sources of pain in the consultation, rather than immediately resorting to a highly invasive and painful surgery that requires a lengthy healing period? I have tried unsuccessfully to locate a specific mandate from OHIP that photographs should be included as a part of the process to justify insurance coverage since I had never heard of photographs being taken for breast reduction surgeries (with the exception of inclusion in a portfolio of surgical work, but this specialist was not Tonya's surgeon). I was baffled by the function of these photographs. Indeed, they seemed to serve the purpose of highlighting that Tonya's surgery was being performed for purely aesthetic reasons, and perhaps indirectly as a means to assure authority.

Tonya imagined the fate of the photographs as follows: The specialist "had to take some pictures of me, like front and side, and ... those pictures then get sent to some kind of ... review panel, to see whether or not it would actually be covered by OHIP ... I don't know who the panel is made up of. In my memory, it was like [a] faceless panel of doctors." Tonya continued:

> This review committee then basically is looking at your breasts ... Which I thought was totally fascinating and obviously very degrading, it didn't really matter what the notes were what mattered so much was that the actual photos were there, which it shouldn't, it shouldn't and so she sends that off, and then they meet, I don't know how often, and then um, and then she got back in touch with, with me to say yeah it was approved, it would be covered by OHIP.

Tonya's story of the photographs that the specialist took in order to obtain insurance coverage emphasized Tonya's lack of agency and alienation. Part of this stems from having to prove to the state that a cosmetic surgery is in fact necessary, but a substantial part of it is also related to these photographs. Tonya never had an opportunity to see these photographs, and when I asked her if she considered requesting them at the time, she answered, "I'd love to – that would be great. But again I didn't even know that I could, I didn't know that I could ask, that I should, or anything. And, and I wish that I had known that kind of stuff, because it would have been really interesting." One possible reason Tonya felt she had no right to request to see these photographs is that they were permeated with state authority and thus off-limits to her. Although the state photograph is a likeness of the individual, it is an exemplar of objectification of the individual for others. Because Tonya was seeking state-funded insurance, she was particularly obliged to submit to whatever photographic practices the specialist suggested. I question the need for these photographs in order to complete the application for coverage, based on my research of OHIP policies that indicate that the surgeon's professional opinion is the most important consideration, but the power given to the photograph as arbiter in Tonya's narrative is structured by surface imagination.

Since Tonya had never revealed her breasts to anyone in full light before, the process of photographing her breasts so that an anonymous panel could review the photographs was, in her words, "degrading." She understood the photographic evidence as the primary criterion by which this panel would make their decision, even though she had been obliged to give extensive (false) statements about the amount of pain she experienced as a result of her large breasts. Because Tonya expressed a feminist consciousness, she understood that the panel's decision was not necessarily an objective one, but one based on contemporary ideals of women's breasts. It is interesting to note that the majority of these breast ideals are produced photographically through digital manipulation or old-fashioned airbrushing, and that the jury of experts who assessed Tonya's breasts did not assess her breasts in the flesh, so to speak: they made their decisions based on photographs.

Diana's surgeon also took photographs. Diana was photographed three times: before her liposuction, immediately following the surgery, and at the one-month follow-up appointment.[25] The narrative that Diana told about these photographs was markedly different from Tonya's, because Diana was able to see the surgeon's photographs and was untroubled by the fact that the surgeon took photographs. I suggest that these differences may stem from the fact that Tonya's surgery was covered by provincial health insurance and Diana's surgery was performed in the private health care sector: she paid for her surgery herself. Because Tonya had never considered a breast reduction prior to the "boob specialist" suggesting it, it is possible that if the surgery had not been funded by provincial health care, Tonya would have been less willing to undergo the procedure.[26] Tonya's surgical experience happened more in the context of what Davis calls the welfare model of medicine, so she needed to demonstrate a serious medical or psychological problem in order to have surgery. Diana's experience, on the other hand, was fully in the realm of what Davis calls the market model of medicine, where she selected her surgeon independently as a consumer decision. While the surgeon's nurse did say that they would not perform liposuction on her thighs, it is not clear whether this was because thigh liposuction was thought of as unnecessary or because of the high likelihood of an unsatisfactory outcome (dips and lumps in the skin, for example). Tonya found the process of being photographed questionable and degrading, while Diana did not seem to question the process of taking photographs during her appointments with the surgeon and her nurse.

While the surgeon's photographs of Diana's body serve documentary functions, since her surgery took place in the private sector of medicine, this evidence was possibly more important for Diana than it was for her surgeon (or it was important for her surgeon for reasons other than justifying a surgery to an insurance body). If Diana were unsatisfied with the outcomes of her surgery, her complaint would take the form of a consumer complaint against the provider of a product or service for not receiving the full value or quality of a product or service that was promised. Her surgeon stored all the photographs of Diana's body on her computer, and they were able to look at them at every appointment. In this way, the photographs are evidence that the liposuction was successful: Diana could see at each appointment how her body was different, and also how the swelling that occurs after liposuction (which is sometimes quite substantial) lessens over time. This could contribute to Diana's greater consumer satisfaction with the operation, since she had only four pounds of fat removed, a change that might be difficult to notice otherwise. Also, should Diana be unsatisfied with the outcome of her liposuction, the surgeon could use these photographs to assess whether this dissatisfaction is justified.[27] If it is justified, the surgeon could offer a reduced rate or *gratis* follow-up surgery; if unjustified, the surgeon could argue that the patient's expectations were unrealistic. In the latter case, the medical photograph could possibly travel into the legal system as evidence not for insurance purposes, but for a lawsuit.[28]

Tigerlily had a markedly different story about her surgeon's use of photographs. The photographs that her surgeon took during the consultation appointment were not for his own files, nor were they used to demonstrate the efficacy of the surgery. Her surgeon used a photograph of her face as a reference point during the surgery. Presumably the surgeon wanted this photograph because when a person is under general anaesthesia, all the facial muscles relax, so it would be harder to know how the patient's face would look under ordinary circumstances. Tigerlily told a fascinating story about this photograph, which she did not see until the day of the surgery:

He took photographs, and I remember I saw this photograph, I don't think I saw, no, I didn't see the photographs at that consultation

but when I was just going under, just before the surgery, I saw that
photograph and I looked absolutely hideous (laughs) ... You know
I think it seemed to me, it was black and white, it could have been
colour, I think it was black and white but, and ah, it was, like you
were under [inaudible] lights with every, every flaw exposed and
the most unflattering shadows prominent.

This "hideous" photograph, which exposed all of Tigerlily's flaws, was
the last thing she remembers seeing before her surgery. Once again, Tigerlily makes reference to the importance of lighting in her perception of the
attractiveness of her face: the lighting in the surgeon's photograph casts
"unflattering shadows" and displays every imperfection. Succumbing to
general anaesthesia was a kind of relief for Tigerlily from looking at this
grotesque photograph, which held the expectation that she would awake
with a face that no longer resembled the photograph. It is also significant
that although she casts doubt on her memory, Tigerlily remembered the
surgeon's photograph as black and white, not colour. Her remembrance
of the surgeon's photograph as black and white can be thought of in two
ways. First, if we probe the connection between black and white photography and state identification and fine art photography, an authority is automatically conferred on the surgeon's photograph. Until relatively recently
in Canada, all photographs on documents like licences and passports were
black and white,[29] so the surgeon's black and white photograph can be
read in relation to these identification photographs as an unbiased representative of Tigerlily's face. The fine art photograph takes its authority
from so-called high culture, so the black and white photograph can also
be associated with a particular economic value.

Second, the black and white photograph can be seen as representative
of historical photography, rather than state photography, in Tigerlily's
narrative. Making the connection between the surgeon's photograph and
historical photography means that the photographed face that Tigerlily
saw immediately before she went under general anaesthesia is situated
firmly in her past. Like the faded and torn archival photograph, the surgeon's photograph of Tigerlily was a representative of an earlier period
that no longer existed in her narrative. As she lost consciousness, Tigerlily
took one final, ephemeral look backward at the face she was about to

defeat through surgery, and she looked forward to a time when she would no longer face the flaws and "unflattering shadows" that age left across her face.

Each of the photographs discussed above operated as a reminder and evidence for the patient or surgeon. For Tonya, Diana, and Tigerlily, these medical evidence photographs depicted their bodies in an undesirable manner that they sought to ameliorate through surgery. I have outlined the social and cultural implications of before and after photographs in cosmetic surgery, and so far I have argued that cosmetic surgery relies on these photographs specifically in order to sustain the practice through the production and evaluation of these photographic surfaces.

Before and After

The documentary use of photography for the cosmetic surgery profession has been significant and pervasive, but before and after photographs offer documentary proof of only a particularly sanitized, surface imagination version of the surgical story. To put it in more explicit terms, the photographs that are most commonly used to record cosmetic surgery expunge the "surgical" component entirely, and it is impossible to tell if the alteration has occurred through changes to the body or changes to the photograph. The before photographs that I have discussed thus far belong to the interviewees only insofar as they are likenesses of their faces and bodies. However, before and after photographs appear in a wide array of formats, and represent a particularly North American conceptualization of identity. This is a surface imagination conceptualization that is not fixed and can be transformed according to the individual's free will. In fact, the reason there are so many variations on the before and after photograph is that this surface imagination account of identity is so prevalent. Before and after photographs may be found anywhere: in a family album, in medical and state records, in a women's magazine, or on a surgeon's website.

Websites are one of the easiest and most accessible ways to peruse before and after photographs. It is possible to look at a large array of photographs of all types of cosmetic surgery, and to do so privately. This is in contrast to photographs of cosmetic surgery procedures in magazines because magazine articles frequently focus on an individual's story and include only a select number of photographs. Magazine articles, however, have the advantage of offering a narrative of cosmetic surgery that accompanies the photographs, resembling the narration of an album of snapshots. While the Internet abounds with photographic documentation of cosmetic surgery, these photographs usually do not have a story attached to them – the image speaks for itself.[30] However, Internet photographs of cosmetic surgery do provide access to a vast range of surgical outcomes, from successful to disastrous, previously unavailable to potential and actual recipients of cosmetic surgery.

Both Melinda and Leah reviewed before and after photographs of other surgical outcomes on their surgeons' websites. Leah considered these photographs to be confirmation that she had made a good decision. Referring to her initial difficulty in convincing herself that she had made a smart choice, she said, "You really don't know, you don't know what's accurate, unless you're on his website, with his pictures, with his whatever, you really don't know." Here Leah is discussing the possibility that surgeons have vastly differing skill levels (rather than the reality that surgeons operate on vastly differing skins and bodies), and that it is impossible to tell whether you have chosen a good surgeon unless you have had an opportunity to view photographs of his work. Before and after photography on a doctor's website, as conceptualized by Leah, provides public confirmation of her surgeon's skill level and operates as an advertisement for his services. Because her initial appointment with her surgeon was so brief and unsatisfying, Leah took further steps – perusing his self-marketing and making another appointment – to ensure that she was making an informed decision.

Melinda described a different reaction to her surgeon's website. Melinda experienced great conflict about her decision to undergo a breast augmentation operation because of her feminist and leftist politics, as well as her identity as the mother of a girl. She was torn: on the one hand, Melinda felt that larger breasts had once belonged to her, but that they had been taken away; on the other, she was more than aware of the overvaluation and sexualization of large breasts in North American society that demeans many women. She was concerned that her breasts might become the main point of visual attention to her body, and that her daughter might unrealistically compare herself visually to Melinda's body as she matured. These concerns might stem from the surfeit of cultural images of very thin, white, and large breasted women who, generally speaking, are large-breasted due to breast implants. These images have two consequences: first, women who are depicted in, or resemble, these images are rendered anonymous and silent because we think we know what their personalities and lives are like; and second, once a woman considers getting breast implants, these images of augmented women are conjured up. Melinda apparently struggled with these consequences, since she directly expressed a fear of being lumped in with "bubble-headed" women after her surgery, and she indirectly expressed anxiety about having a body that is anonymous and generic.

Her surgeon's website, and particularly the before and after photos section, alleviated several of Melinda's fears. She said, "I think it also helped looking on the website, at the different pictures of women who had gone and you know, what they had done, and that other people did look like, how I looked, and some of them actually were large-breasted, where they just wanted to make themselves perkier, or what have you, and all kinds of different bodies, right?" While Melinda felt uncomfortable during the consultation appointment (which was perhaps an extension of her general discomfort about the procedure), when she went home and looked at photographs on the surgeon's website, she felt reassured. Melinda was particularly interested in women who looked like her, and women with large breasts (who presumably did not look like her). The photographs of women who looked like her offered visual proof that not all women who seek out breast implants are seeking very large breasts, and also that it is not unusual for women with bodies similar to hers to want implants. The photographs of large-breasted women who underwent breast lift procedures provided a counterpoint to the breast augmentations, in that those photographs demonstrated to Melinda that dissatisfaction with one's breasts is primarily an individual phenomenon. Because it is possible to be dissatisfied with one's large breasts, even though large breasts are culturally valued, Melinda became more convinced of the role of psychological explanations for breast surgeries and emphasized these explanations over social explanations, although we might well see these two kinds of explanation as impossible to disentangle. In the context of the photographs that appeared on the surgeon's website, Melinda's decision became more and more acceptable to her because breast surgery was visually proven to be no longer a surgery that only one type of body receives (in this case, small-breasted women). Instead, "all kinds of different bodies" might seek out breast surgery, for individualized and psychological yet visually oriented reasons that are generally inaccessible to the viewer of the photograph. Melinda's experience of the before and after story on the surgeon's website was quite different from Leah's, who used these photographs to assess the skill of the surgeon to whom she has been referred. While Leah's narrative can be thought of as seeing a similar before and after story in each of the photographs (a success story that emerges through the surgeon's expertise), Melinda saw multiple before and after stories (stories that emerge from differing experiences of breastedness). Rather than serving as evidence of the surgeon's skill, the before and after photographs had a normalizing function in Melinda's narrative of her breast augmentation.

So far, the before and after photographs I have discussed share territory with medical evidence photography; but they also carry over into the realm of advertising. They provide proof of the surgeon's skills to the public and have a normalizing effect on cosmetic surgical procedures. We also trust these images in a way that we do not trust many other images in cultural circulation. We might be skeptical of the *choice* of photographs, assuming that the surgeon would place only the most successful surgeries on her website. However, we are less likely to be suspicious of the *content* of the photographs, since we have faith that the photographs have in no way been retouched or otherwise manipulated because they are presented as documentation of a professional's practice. If we were to distrust the content of the photographs, they would not have the same reassuring effect.

There is, however, another category of before and after photography that is slightly more suspect, but can be nonetheless very important for those seeking out cosmetic surgery. Women's magazines are a popular source of information on cosmetic surgery, as I explored in chapter 2. They not only offer photographic material about cosmetic surgery, but they also incorporate personal narratives that overlay the photographs, as well as advice from medical experts. However, women's magazines are notorious culprits in the production, distribution, and promotion of unrealistic images of women's bodies. Indeed, the publication of stories about cosmetic surgery could be considered one of a plethora of techniques that women's magazines employ to nourish body-hating attitudes – alongside diet and exercise tips; digitally manipulated photographs of already extremely thin women modelling clothing, makeup, and accessories; and advertising images. Unlike the photographs on a surgeon's website, photographs in women's magazines are not deemed trustworthy. Both Tigerlily and Nicanor discussed women's magazines in their narratives, but in different ways. It is interesting that Tigerlily and Nicanor, who both underwent cosmetic surgeries that aimed to address the aging of their faces, discussed women's magazines, which proscribe bodies outside of a very thin, white ideal and bodies that are more than twenty years old.

Tigerlily had her surgery in 1997, approximately ten years before we met. Historically, this is the period immediately before the contemporary cosmetic surgery boom as an industry and in popular culture. At the time of her surgery, there were no television shows that focused on cosmetic surgery, and lunchtime procedures like Botox and other injections were not featured prominently in popular culture. Her surgery happened in the wake of several silicone implant lawsuits in the United States; and silicone implants were banned in Canada, except in extraordinary circumstances usually related to post-mastectomy reconstruction.[31] In this context, women's magazines were a major source of information about cosmetic surgery. Tigerlily's narrative attested to this:

> I didn't really know what to expect, what helped me make the decision finally was a magazine article which I had kept maybe for a year or two, in one of the women's magazines. And it was a relation by a woman who had been through a face-lift, she had a couple of full-face photographs, I think a before and an after and after the surgery, and she had bandages, and anyway there was some good photographs and it was the most explicit [way of] relating of the process, that I'd ever seen, and that was actually quite comforting. You know actually, the not knowing what to expect can be very anxiety provoking.

As noted earlier, Tigerlily was emphatic that her story was "not ... dramatic" in contrast to "other women," and she said that she did not experience a great deal of pain or other discomfort after her surgery.[32] However, her anxieties appeared to lie in the unknowns of the surgery, because while she was realistic in that she did not "expect to come out looking like a teenager," she didn't really know what her face would look like after surgery. In Tigerlily's narrative, the women's magazine article served a reassuring purpose similar to the surgeons' websites for Leah and Melinda, although again in a slightly different fashion. The article demystified face-lift surgeries for Tigerlily, and the specific component that was most reassuring was the photographic narrative of the face-lift. Tigerlily said nothing about the textual narrative that accompanied the article, and instead said that the photographs were the "most explicit" that she had seen. She said that the "full-face photographs" depicted "a before and an after and an after the surgery," which I interpreted as adding a step that is frequently erased in before and after photograph: the in-between stage of healing. Through these photographs, Tigerlily was able to imagine what face-lift surgery would look like immediately following the procedure, and after the healing process was over, and she used the medium of the photograph of another woman's face to do so. Here the photograph was a promise of what surgery can accomplish, and through inclusion in a women's magazine, cosmetic surgery was less threatening and placed firmly within the constellation of practices that are used to maintain a normative feminine body.

In part through the inspiration of this magazine article, Tigerlily decided to photographically document her cosmetic surgery and healing process:

> T – so I basically, I took a photograph of myself every day 'cause, I think I mentioned that in my notes, and I don't know whether I threw them out or not because I never really looked at them again, nobody I know is interested!
> R – Right!
> T – I would have been interested, I think if I did, known somebody to do that before I made my decision.

I communicated more extensively with Tigerlily by email before our first meeting than I did with the other participants. When she mentioned that she had taken many photographs throughout her process, I asked if I could look at them during the interview.[33] Tigerlily decided to imitate the format of the before and after magazine story that she so appreciated, and she never shared these photographs with anyone because "nobody [she] knows is interested." Thinking about this comment alongside

Tigerlily's comment that in her social circles cosmetic surgery is discussed as a possibility every year after a woman turns fifty, and yet actual surgeries are definitely not talked about, poses a noteworthy contradiction in the narrative. In a social group that discussed cosmetic surgery every year after turning fifty, how is it possible that no one wanted to see Tigerlily's photographs? Is this because of lack of interest, or is it because Tigerlily had not discussed her surgery with friends who had not had surgery themselves? The photographs that Tigerlily took after her surgery seem to belong more to Tigerlily's healing process than to form part of a supplement to her narrative of cosmetic surgery or serve as an aid for friends who might be considering cosmetic surgery. These images are not idealized, as they might be if they appeared in a women's magazine, but are instead a quotidian account of Tigerlily's surgery that enabled her to look at her face objectively and sensibly, a practice that seemed important for Tigerlily's understanding of her face-lift narrative.

I conclude these accounts of the actual cosmetic surgery photographs that the participants discussed with a brief mention of Nicanor's understanding of the effects of the idealized images contained in women's magazines. Nicanor understood one effect of women's magazines to be that women's value is measured in their appearances, "because nobody says, you know, forget it, I look like a witch, but I'm very smart." Nicanor considered herself complicit in this action; although she thought that this is wrong and "shouldn't be this way ... it is and nobody does anything really, to change it." She was troubled by her own judgmental looking practices when reading a fashion magazine, admitting to looking at photographs of models and thinking to herself, "My god, these people are very ugly! What, you know, why are they here?"

Nicanor's first response to the photographs she saw in magazines is symptomatic of a larger set of psychical responses to the image, and in a broad North American cultural context, particularly images of women. An almost automatic response to images of women in magazines is to assess them against a fantasmatic, non-existent idealized woman who is a composite of previous images of women that have themselves been retouched and manipulated. What might prompt Nicanor's response to the model? Perhaps it was the expectation that models embody an impossible ideal, or that a magazine image be digitally altered to suit this ideal, or even that the model herself ought to be altered through surgery prior to being photographed for the magazine. I would suggest that these responses are not as separate as this list indicates, but rather they intimate that the transient logic of the photograph and the transformative logic of cosmetic surgery are so prevalent that our processes of looking at an image in a magazine conflate these expectations into one. If we combine this suggestion with the easy familiarity that we have with the photographic image, it makes sense that the photograph has alternately offered evidential value, inspirational material, and comforting hope to the interviewees.

Conclusion

Silverman's theory of the idealized image, in conjunction with Parveen Adams's consideration of the image emptied of meaning, sheds light on the detrimental and productive cultural effects of the photograph in cosmetic surgery. Silverman observes that American and French feminist theorists assume that women are more intimately connected with their bodies than are men. This, of course, has to do with the familiar occidental binaries of man/woman and mind/body, the condition that women are charged with the principal responsibility for the care and maintenance of other bodies, and other more biologically essentialist claims involving the centrality of menstruation, pregnancy, childbirth, and lactation to women's life experiences. Moving in a contrasting direction, feminists have charged others (particularly men) with essentializing women and associating women primarily with their bodies. Freudian and Lacanian psychoanalysis is a popular target for such critiques, and many feminist theorists have been particularly critical of the concept of castration. This feminist understanding of castration deems that psychoanalysis automatically condemns women to inferiority due to their lack of a penis, whereas men are endowed with superiority via their possession of a penis. This reading, however, is itself predicated on biological essentialism; while it is valid to question Freud's choice of "penis" as the signifier for desire (indeed, Lacan's modification of the penis into the phallus is an attempt – more or less effective, depending on one's perspective – to circumvent this biological equivalence), the concept of castration as the opening up of a lack at the heart of our being is fundamental to psychoanalytic theory. It is crucial here to think of castration not as a physical threat or fact (as in the Freudian story of the woman as castrated, or the boy fearing that the father will cut off his penis), but rather as a metaphor for the inability of language to express our interior life, including emotions and thoughts, as well as the limitations that are imposed on us from the Symbolic. Castration is our entrance (regardless of whether we are sexed male or female at birth) into the Symbolic realm of language and law, and the consequence of language as insufficient to hold our psychical life. We are all castrated, and without the loss occasioned by castration there could be no desire.

Silverman challenges the assumption that women are more intimately connected to their bodies than men because it does not take into account the cultural fabrication of the body. The assumption holds women to be naive readers of images who consider the image to be the same as their being. Of the castration crisis in the girl, Silverman says,

> The castration crisis can perhaps best be understood as the moment at which the young female subject first apprehends herself no longer within the pleasurable frame of the original maternal imago, but within the radically deidealizing screen or cultural image-repertoire, which makes of her body the very image of "lack." To be more precise, the castration crisis is synonymous with the moment at which the girl first feels herself *seen* in ways that are in radical excess of her negative Oedipal relation to her mother, and which are not those which she would choose for herself. She is – as a consequence – held to an identification which she would otherwise refuse.[34]

This passage speaks of an entry into the Symbolic dimensions of femininity through the Imaginary images of women that the girl is confronted with. The girl is culturally compelled to identify with de-idealizing images and at the same time she is identified by others with these images. The consequence is an identification with lack in order to assimilate to a normative femininity. Silverman argues that women are "exhorted over and over again to aspire to the ideal of the exceptional woman, the woman whose extravagant physical beauty miraculously erases marks of castration."[35] Here feminine beauty functions to cover over the female subject's castration through visual cues that phallically encase her in the protective armour of beauty. Exceptional beauty is a means for the female subject to simultaneously maintain her lack and yet remain as its inverse so that the male subject can continue to occupy the ruse of having the phallus and the female subject can be the phallus that can sustain his desire. The possibility of embodying exceptional beauty is a type of contradictory panacea for castration that positions the female subject in what Silverman names a "double bind" in which she is directed to manifest something she is barred from becoming.

Silverman identifies narcissistic object-choice as yet another potential protest of the female subject's "forced identification with lack."[36] This is epitomized in "that unrequited love which many women direct toward the images of ideal femininity which they are exhorted to approximate, but prohibited from replicating. Significantly, this vain but nonetheless imperative quest after absolute beauty has nothing to do with self-love; it is predicated on the impossibility of loving the self. Only an imaginary union with the desired image would make possible a 'jubilant' self-apprehension, but that image remains at an irreducible remove."[37]

The relation to the images of ideal femininity discussed by Silverman can be explained through two manifestations of narcissistic self-love articulated by Freud: loving that which we might like to become, and loving someone who can love the subject in order to make up for the "impossibility of loving the self." The second manifestation is "passive" according to Silverman, and requires the subject to think of herself as love object for another, which creates the conditions for a compensatory self-love.[38] The first manifestation, in contrast, is "active" and involves cross-gendered identification and love of someone who "represents 'the narcissistic ideal of the man whom [she] had wished to become.'"[39] This is an escape from the radical impossibility of being the exceptional woman, because it enables a solution to femininity that does not entrap the female subject. Silverman states explicitly here that she is not arguing against idealization – which is the prerequisite for identificatory and erotic love of the other – but against the manner in which idealization gets tangled up with culturally valorized images and norms.[40]

Lacan argues that we idealize particular bodies over others through the Imaginary register, and because the Imaginary is the register of spectacle and display, idealizations are formed in the visual field. In *Seminar VII: The Ethics of Psychoanalysis,* Lacan states that "society takes some comfort from the mirages that moralists, artists, artisans, designers of dresses and hats, and creators of imaginary forms in general supply it with."[41] These comforting fantasies are surface imagination fantasies about swathing the body and its environs in transformative surfaces, and as Kaja Silverman argues, they are fantasies that lead to some bodies being valued and desired more than others.[42] The images that appear in photographs, as an imaginary "textual production," can be thought of as stirring the same fantasies that Lacan invokes. As the photograph is retouched, and the subject of the photograph is operated upon, the surgical body comes to be the culturally idealized body (whether those corporeal alterations occur by surgery or not).

Further, Lacan also argues through his conceptualization of the screen that we have little control over how our bodies are seen by others. In contrast to the mirror, whose image bears a resemblance to the baby, the screen does not reflect anything and thus does not bear any indexical relationship to the subject who is represented by the screen. The screen bears the weight of idealizing and de-idealizing representations, determined not by the individual's look but the cultural gaze as symbolic and de-subjectivized. Consequently, we are determined by how the cultural gaze regards our bodies.[43] Thus, fantasies of corporeal disintegration emerge when the subject realizes that the ideal imago is forever unattainable,[44] and also that only certain subjects have flattering cultural representations of their bodies with which to identify.[45]

I have linked together these two insights because they are crucial to understanding the relationship between photography and cosmetic surgery. Being shown images of culturally idealized bodies confronts the ego with the reality that, culturally speaking, the external representation of the body (bodily ego) is unlovable. This summons fantasies of bodily disintegration, which, as I have already argued, shares the same fragmentary logic and fantasy as cosmetic surgery and photography. Cosmetic surgery offers the ego a method of dealing with the impossibility of even coming close to the ideal imago, and the visual evidence and inspiration promised by photography strengthens this method. The surface imagination fantasies of cosmetic surgery promise a wholeness and a control in the face of the impossibility of the ideal imago.

Lacan characterizes the camera as the explanatory vehicle for the gaze, because the camera makes us aware that we are being seen and produces an illusion of what others see through the photograph. In each of the in-

terviewee's narratives of individual photographs, the photograph as a document of "being seen" was a prevalent theme. Tonya's narrative is an exemplar of this notion because her breasts (which had never before been
seen in full light) were photographed and the images were sent to an
anonymous panel to be scrutinized and evaluated. Even in the narratives
about looking at photographs in magazines and on websites, the interviewees are imagining how their own bodies will be seen after surgery
using the visual evidence offered by the photographs. In order to think
through some of the implications of the camera's de-subjectivized gaze
for cosmetic surgery, I want to return to a rather eccentric example of
cosmetic surgery and photography, an example that nevertheless illuminates the fragmentation of the idealized feminine body by photography
and cosmetic surgery, and also reveals something about the stories that
before and after photography is allowed to tell. I want to conclude by
considering Adams's insightful discussion of the feminine body as empty
image. The discussion of an extraordinary case – French performance
artist ORLAN – offers a synthesis of the effects of thinking of the body
photographically outlined in this chapter.

The French performance artist ORLAN reproduces, explores, and
exploits the conventions of photography in cosmetic surgery in her
surgical performances. The performances are, moreover, a critique of
masculinist values of authorship and originality in art history. ORLAN's
use of photographic evidence disrupts and extends vernacular cosmetic
surgery photographs by presenting the viewer with the interstices between
before and after, showing the elided content much desired by potential
recipients of cosmetic surgery, and offering an example of how vernacular
and art photography might be put into conversation and tension with
one another. ORLAN's work has offered a sustained critique of feminine
beauty norms throughout her career, and "The Reincarnation of Saint-
ORLAN" uses cosmetic surgery as a means to transgress feminine beauty
precisely by invoking the censored content that occurs between the before
and the after photographs.

ORLAN's body of work has critiqued representations of feminine beauty
in Western art for over thirty-five years, often tackling the issues of identity
and embodiment with lucid insight and sharp humour.[46] ORLAN has experimented with a variety of media and has been particularly preoccupied with the impact of technology on art and the body, as well as

psychoanalytic theories of femininity. "The Reincarnation of Saint-
ORLAN" is a multi-stage, multi-media, and interdisciplinary series of surgical performances that employs analogue and digital photography to
record the performances and enact further alterations to ORLAN's body.
Peggy Phelan refers to this conglomeration of surgery and photography
as "photographic sculpture,"[47] a phrase I love because it captures the ambiguity of the images of ORLAN's body. Her goal is the radical transformation of her body, but this is not a goal in a conventional sense, for this
goal has no end; as Jill O'Bryan suggestively writes, "there is no before
and after."[48] O'Bryan makes the point that ORLAN's body, like all our
bodies, is in a constant state of becoming something else.

However, I would like to twist O'Bryan's statement to argue that
ORLAN's work does something more radical: it literalizes the violent
processes through which normative femininity and sexual difference are
produced in surface imagination cultures. The visual objectification of the
body and discussion of photographs offered by the interviewees are an
interesting contrast to ORLAN's project because they do not use visual
language to suggest a body that is in the process of becoming. Rather,
they use visual language in order to describe a particular *moment* of becoming, after which their bodies were able to feel more stable, and less
contingent, as discussed in the last chapter.

ORLAN's surgical project is to appropriate features of feminine images
in Western art history, specifically DaVinci's Mona Lisa, Botticelli's Venus,
Moreau's Europa, Gérard's Psyche, and the Fontainebleu School's Diana.
These figures are not chosen for the specific aesthetic value of the feature
to be surgically created, but because of their mythical and fantastic qualities, and the piecing together of these figures in one body suggests the
fragmented and contradictory nature of femininity that is disavowed in
Western art in favour of the unified and whole image. Indeed, while
ORLAN selects feminine icons in Western art history for inspiration, she
manipulates this decision through her idiosyncratic choices of features to
appropriate: for example, while it is the smile of the Mona Lisa that is
legendary, ORLAN instead opts to emulate the temples on Mona Lisa's
brow. The piecing together of these facial fragments enacts the process of
composite photography upon the skin. During the surgical performances
of "The Reincarnation of Saint- ORLAN" (which occurred in the 1990s),
ORLAN remained conscious, which is again a disruptive opening up of

the in-between space of the surgical field. The operating theatre comes to life in its status as a site of drama: the surgeons and the artist are clothed in couture costumes, a soundtrack adds dramatic flair, ORLAN's work is hung and projected onto the walls as a set, and ORLAN reads her own writing and psychoanalytic texts as scripts. ORLAN situates her voice at the level of the camera's gaze, and by narrating the performance as though she were an impassive observer rather than the operated upon body, confounds the relation between subject and object of the image. Her performances were photographed, filmed, and broadcast to world art centres, and we might think of these performances as illuminating the forgotten interstices between before and after photographs.

ORLAN's photograph titled "Women Resemble the Moon, My Eyes Resemble Flowers, or Self-Portrait with Narcissus Produced by the Body-Machine Six Days after the Seventh Surgery Performance" fascinates me for its refusal to be assimilated into the social and cultural surface imagination discourses of cosmetic surgery. ORLAN faces directly into the camera, following the conventions of the after photograph exactly and even improving on it through staging the glorious surgical triumph like a beauty pageant by using the cosmopolitan backdrop and flowers. However, consider this photograph in contrast to the before and after photographs of face and eye lift patients from *Harper's Bazaar* and a cosmetic surgeon's website, presented in the previous chapter (Figures 2.4 and 2.5). Having cosmetic surgery on one's face and eyes makes one look as though she has been "punched in the face," to use Nicanor's words. In the conventions of before and after photographs, this "punched in the face" stage is censored and what we see could just as easily have been achieved with a computer cursor. And indeed, only Tigerlily touches on this "punched in the face" stage through the photographs she took of herself during the surgery as well as the photographs in the magazine article that helped her decided to undergo cosmetic surgery. Notably, Tigerlily does not describe the content of these in-between photographs, even though she describes the before photograph in all its unflattering detail.

Returning to the photograph at hand, notice that ORLAN does not smile into the camera. Instead she looks into it with an ambiguous expression that might be longing, disinterest, or even lust. As the viewer, we don't know and we cannot know because we are not the photograph's subject. ORLAN's documentary use of photography in her art rejects the

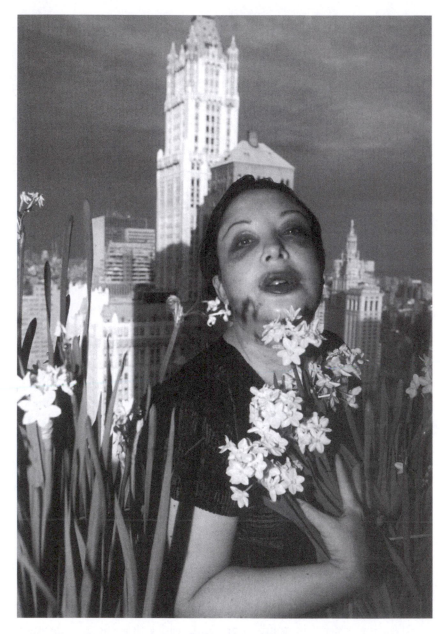

3.1 ORLAN, 27 November 1993, "Women Resemble the Moon, My Eyes Resemble Flowers, or Self-Portrait with Narcissus Produced by the Body-Machine Six Days after the Seventh Surgery-Performance"

covering up of the truly remarkable healing phase, and presents it as victoriously as the standard after photograph is presented on surgeons' websites and women's magazines. She expresses the bloodiness, the horror, and the joy of literally opening the body and altering it through surgery, and in some ways challenges the social obligation to keep cosmetic surgery private and secret. Her evocation of narcissism in psychoanalytic theory as well as the myth and representation of Narcissus in Western art history through the flowers provocatively engages with the debate about whether cosmetic surgery is pursued for external vanity reasons or internal psychological reasons. ORLAN has remarked that as a child and young woman, she did not recognize her mirror image as herself, quite unlike Narcissus.[49] Kate Ince argues that ORLAN's art reverses the process of cosmetic surgery since ORLAN is not trying to ameliorate her appearance to fit beauty standards; rather, she is trying to transform her body to fit with her artistic vision, even though doing this makes her appearance less in conformity with feminine beauty standards, as the photographs reveal.[50]

I propose that while "The Reincarnation of Saint- ORLAN" is an interdisciplinary project, it follows a photographic surface imagination logic, a logic that is shared with the cosmetic surgery profession. This logic considers the body to be in pieces that can be posed, positioned, cut, augmented, or retouched according to the photographer or surgeon's wishes and skills. While the profession of cosmetic surgery promises a transformation of the body using the medium of photography as a support, due to the contingency of the flesh, it cannot mimic the magic of photography and thus cannot wholly deliver on the promises it makes. ORLAN's work highlights the contingency and vulnerability of the body, linking the masculinism of Western art history with cosmetic surgery and hyperbolizing the hidden carnal and psychical violence that creates feminine sexual difference that is further obscured by the before and after photograph. ORLAN's photographs of her surgical performances and surgical results literalizes and corporealizes the violence of fragmentation, the impossibility of living up to the idealized feminine body, and the injury that results from being unable to unite the exteroceptive ego with the proprioceptive ego.

Adams argues that the before and after photograph "effect[s] a closure of refiguration."[51] This closure is necessary, she states, because many find it difficult to accept the notion of a face (and I would add, a body) that is not original and not in pursuit of a final image.[52] This is a contradictory closure, since a psychic wish for finality and stability conflicts with the postmodern ideal of endless transformation. ORLAN's oeuvre is difficult for audiences to tolerate, and incites interrogation about her psychological well-being because it lays bare the fundamental promises of cosmetic surgery about the ethical responsibility of the surgeons who operate on her body.

Adams suggestively observes that ORLAN "is an image trapped in the body of a woman."[53] This insinuates a common axiom of transsexuality in the popular imagination that is appropriated by cosmetic surgery, which is that transsexual surgeries are justified and understandable when the individual expresses that they feel trapped in the wrong body.[54] The alignment of the exteroceptive with the proprioceptive ego offers the same explanation. Do we not also see the image trapped in the body in all narratives of cosmetic surgery? ORLAN dissolves the debate about whether woman is born or made, according to Adams, since for ORLAN, "being a woman is dependent on continuously being born through surgery."[55] ORLAN conceptualizes herself as image, forever watched by the cultural gaze, and exposes the pervasiveness of the surgical order that indeed demands that our understanding of women be conceived through a surgical-photographic eye. Adams argues that ORLAN's work challenges the completeness that the cosmetic surgery industry aspires to, which is true to an extent but is not the whole story. While Adams's statement that the body is "unfinished"[56] until it has undergone cosmetic surgery is indeed an accurate summary of the *promise* of cosmetic surgery, the *reality* of cosmetic surgery is that once you have had surgery, it is almost inevitable that you will have more surgery either as additional surgeries, corrective surgeries, or maintenance surgeries. Thus cosmetic surgeries in themselves render the body "unfinished."

ORLAN's work is disturbing not because it is in opposition to "ordinary" cosmetic surgery in its fragmented state of incompletion; it horrifies because it exposes just how unfinished *all* cosmetic surgery really is. While I agree with Adams that cosmetic surgery holds out a "narcissistic optimism" that is not present in ORLAN's surgical performances,[57] the absence of this optimism is also *horrifying* in ORLAN's photographic and video representations of her performances. ORLAN's photographs empty the image of the idealized feminine body of its meaning through the detachment of her face to reveal that there is nothing but raw, bloody flesh behind it. As in the cosmetic surgery profession, the photograph is engaged precisely because it effects the impartial distance between the viewer and the operated upon body. ORLAN's engagement with photographs opens up a space that collapses the distance between the interior and exterior of the body, revealing something quite new about surface imagination cultures. This is not the story that before and after photography is authorized to tell according to the surface imagination narratives of the cosmetic surgery industry, which erase the violence done to the body through imagining it as bits and pieces that can be refashioned by the scalpel. ORLAN exposes this violence using the same medium – the photograph – that the cosmetic surgery industry uses as a medium of concealment. Adams suggests that the gap between ORLAN as the voice that narrates throughout the surgery and ORLAN as the object that is sliced by scalpel and pierced by needle is "stark."[58] She concludes her book by saying that "it is not that surgery has transformed [ORLAN], but that surgery has changed our experience of the image."[59] Undeniably. The image and the surgery are indissoluble.

Throughout this chapter, I have argued that the photographic image haunts cosmetic surgery and encourages patients to take the position of the camera's gaze by self-objectifying their bodies as surgical raw material. Photography sustains surface imagination and supports the practice of cosmetic surgery through fragmentation and transformation of the body image. Looking at a body from the perspective of the cosmetic surgeon is much like looking at a body through the lens of the camera; and likewise the photographic editor looks at the body in the same way a surgeon might. Photographs offer inspiration to cosmetic surgery patients, providing many examples of bodily configurations that are desirable in a contemporary context, or they provide evidence of the more desirable past of one's body. Whether an alteration happens through the skin, flesh, and bone or through photo retouching, the effect on the image printed on photographic paper looks the same. Because we in Canada and other Western nations live in a photographically and visually oriented culture, the difference between photo and surgical retouching is negligible. Many, if not most cosmetic surgeries make the body and face look good in clothing and accessories, though underneath the clothes and beyond the hairline the damage to the body becomes apparent. Cosmetic surgery alleviates some degree of psychic suffering, and it does so through the visual realm of the surface by preparing the body for photography. The photographic image is symptomatic of cosmetic surgery's impossible ideal. Photography is the idealized form of surgical intervention because it skims past the corporeal body, which too often interferes with cosmetic surgery, whose surgical interventions into the body's surface produce less than perfect results on the de-idealized surface of cosmetic surgery: the skin.

THE FEMININE SKIN
AS ANXIOUS ARCHIPELAGO

4

Skin is the textile of time and writing. It is the first and enduring medium with which we encounter the world, and skin comes to metaphorically embody the relationship between our interior and exterior lives. The fabric of our skin is able to accomplish a feat that nothing else in our lives is able to, no matter how fervently we may wish – it can turn time backwards. An opening up of the body through blade or fire seals itself, restoring the skin's integrity through a stunning process of scarring and reparation. Steven Connor astutely observes that cosmetic surgery attempts to replicate the magical properties of skin to coax time into dissolution.[1] He offers many metaphorical alternatives to thinking about the skin as a screen or a slate, but his suggestion that the skin can be thought of as an archipelago is a particularly touching metaphor for the skin in cosmetic surgery. In cosmetic surgery, skin is a psychic and somatic archipelago of meaning, experience, and memory, dispersed across a social and cultural sea. As a cartographer of skin in cosmetic surgery, I must persistently attend to this landscape of skin to resist collapsing it into a flat, static surface.

Skin is the earliest interface through which we encounter otherness. This otherness is experienced tactilely, and we continue to experience the self and other as separated by our skins. The skin is racialized, gendered, and sexualized through its reading by others, which marks a shift from the tactility of early infantile experience to the visual experience that predominates our contemporary understandings of skin. Focusing on the skin as cosmetic surgery's de-idealized surface, I elaborate on the psychic promises and difficulties of conceiving one's body according to the terms of surface imaginations. The skin is a troubled surface in contrast to the photograph; it is miraculous in a different way, yet recalcitrant. The restorative and inscriptive capacities of skin sustain the central surface imagination fantasy of cosmetic surgery, which is that we can consider our bodies as infinitely alterable and customizable according to our wishes. An intervention into the skin through cosmetic surgery is a means of asserting agency over the body with the hope of alleviating suffering, although this agency is always partial: the body itself is contingent and may not respond to our interventions.

A psychoanalytic understanding of skin situates the skin's importance to cosmetic surgery, providing a foundation for my analysis of the skin as a de-idealized surface in the interview narratives. I begin with Freud's theory of the bodily ego, which considers how the experiences of the body (and in particular the experiences of otherness) structure the psychic apparatus; this is key to interpreting the way surface imaginations conceptualize the skin. Freud posits that the ego cannot be thought of as a surface, but rather as a *projection* of a surface. This insight is the inspiration for Didier Anzieu's metaphor of the skin ego. The interview narratives trouble and complicate these concepts of the bodily and skin egos through their emphasis on contingency, the relation between the interior and exterior of our bodies, and time.

In contrast to the idealized surface of the photograph, the de-idealized surface of the skin challenges the fantasy that the body can be altered according to our desires in three overlapping ways. First, the skin is a site through which we experience and learn contingency and accident,[2] and thus cosmetic surgery can be thought of as a way of asserting control over the contingent skin. However, having cosmetic surgery also throws the patient into a confrontation with the contingency of skin, for it is impossible to absolutely predict the results of a surgery. Here I explore how participants discussed the unknown and accidental qualities of their skin. Second, skin is an allegory of time, and time is marked upon our bodies. These marks may appear suddenly and temporarily, as in the bruise or laceration, or they may happen gradually and permanently, as in the wrinkle or scar. Here I am concerned with skin transformations and the delineations of time, and I argue that cosmetic surgery facilitates the assumption of a second skin[3] for the patient. And, finally, the skin is a metaphor and locus for the exchange and connection between our interior psychic lives and our exterior social world. The complaint that one does not *feel* on the inside the same way that one *appears* to the outside frequently precipitates a decision to have cosmetic surgery. This complaint, often described as feeling as though one is in the "wrong body," marks an interesting parallel and divergence between "cosmetic" and "sex reassignment" surgeries, and toward the end of the chapter I offer a speculative consideration of this (dis)connection. In conclusion, I consider how the skin is a site where the interior and exterior worlds collide and negotiations between the individual and the cultural occur.

The Bodily Ego and the Unconscious

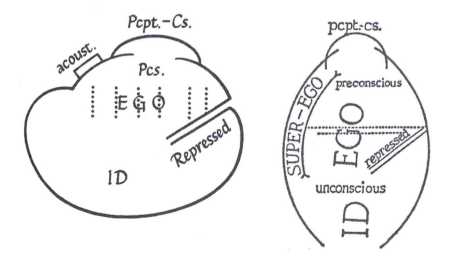

4.1 and 4.2 Two of Sigmund Freud's structural diagrams of the mental apparatus reprinted from "The Ego and the Id" (1923) and "The Dissection of the Psychical Personality" (1933)

Before I discuss Didier Anzieu's lovely metaphor of the skin ego, I want to first trace my path back to Freud's skin-sheathed theories of the unconscious, consciousness, and the ego. In "The Ego and the Id" (1923) Freud explains that the role of the ego is to act as a mediating space between the unconscious (id) and the preconscious-conscious (perception-consciousness system and the external world), and describes the ego as a "frontier-creature"[4] and "a poor creature owing service to three masters and consequently menaced by three dangers: from the external world, from the libido of the id, and from the severity of the superego."[5] The ego's wish is to impress upon the id the demands of the external world, or to assert the dominance of the reality principle over the id's insistent adherence to the pleasure principle and the death drive.

Freud's theory is astonishing in its affirmation that our body is a site of internal and external perceptions and the locus of mental processes, which stands in contrast to the Cartesian privileging of the mind over the body. According to Freud, the manner in which we perceive unconscious mental processes with our consciousness parallels our perception of the external world with our sense organs.[6] He says that the unconscious is timeless, but consciousness, like skin, bears the burden of time.[7] When we touch ourselves, we *see* our bodies as we would see any other object, but the reflexivity of the *touch* relationship gives us an idea of the experience of a location that perceives from the inside and the outside (like the ego): "A person's own body, and above all its surface, is a place from which both external and internal perceptions may spring. It is *seen* like any other object, but to the *touch* it yields two kinds of sensations, one of which might be equivalent to an internal perception."[8] In this way the body is the foundation of our psychical lives, and in particular the skin occupies the ambiguous condition of being a reciprocal organ that feels from the inside and out and, further, can touch itself. When Freud says, "the ego is first and foremost a bodily ego,"[9] he means that the body is inseparable from the mental apparatus and they act as templates of experience for each other. Unlike consciousness (the surface of our mental apparatus), the ego is "not merely a surface entity, but is itself the projection of a surface"[10] because it projects the conscious world to the unconscious and back again in its mediating function. Similarly, the skin is more than surface in its vast communicative capacities between the interior and exterior of the body and between the conscious and unconscious, navigating through a vast topography of embodied thought and feeling.

Freud's description of the ego as a *projection of surface* evokes both the idealized and de-idealized surfaces of cosmetic surgery. The word "projection" can refer to visual technologies that transmit an image onto a flat surface (for example, a slide projector), or it can refer to the psychoanalytic concept of how qualities of one's self are externalized and perceived as qualities of others (both positive and negative). Projecting an image is a literal and figurative action within the surface imaginations of cosmetic surgery; the patient wants to project a more positive or accurate image of herself to the world, and the patient and surgeon rely on the projection of photographic images in order to envision the results of surgery. The negative qualities of the skin are projected outward onto others, who are truly old, fat, or ugly, unlike the patient who is unjustly afflicted by the appearance of being so. The psychical action of cosmetic surgery happens at the level of the ego and the image, and because Freud developed his theory at the historical moment when surface imagination logic emerges, this convergence of the ego, photography, and skin as mediator is no accident.

In a rather peculiar little essay that appears chronologically later than "The Unconscious" and "The Ego and the Id," Freud elaborates his theory of the perceptual system. "A Note upon the Mystic Writing-Pad" (1925) brings Freud's theory of mind into close contact with the skin's surface as a consequence of his selecting the mystic writing-pad as a metaphor to explain perception. The mystic writing-pad is a children's writing toy that has three layers: the top layer is made of strong, transparent celluloid; the middle layer is made of a translucent waxed paper that is fragile and sticks lightly to the bottom layer, composed of brown wax. When you write on the top layer with a stylus as you would write on a piece of paper with a pencil, the middle layer is impressed by the stylus into the bottom wax layer, and the writing appears. Once you decide you would like a fresh writing surface, you simply lift up the top and middle layers to unstick the writing-impressions from the wax. Your writing surface is now clear, and a slight imprint of the writing is left in the wax layer. Like a sheet of paper, the mystic writing-pad is capable of maintaining permanent traces, but it does not have to be replaced once it is full of writing; like the chalkboard, it can be reused endlessly, but without the drawback of losing the traces of writing every time you erase the board to write anew. While the devices that we use to amplify our senses emulate the sense they are to enhance (Freud gives the examples of "spectacles, photographic cameras, ear-trumpets"), he comments that "devices to aid our memory seem particularly imperfect, since our mental apparatus accomplishes precisely what they cannot: it has an unlimited receptive capacity for new perceptions and nevertheless lays down permanent – even though not unalterable – memory-traces of them."[11] Together, the top and middle layers of the mystic writing-pad perform the same function as the perception-consciousness system, taking in traces from the external world but also protecting its own fragility, and the wax layer beneath is analogous to the unconscious, which retains all the traces filtered through the perception-consciousness system.

As Anzieu has noted, "A Note upon the Mystic Writing-Pad" presages later anatomical descriptions of the skin as a membrane composed primarily of two layers that protect the interior of the body: the epidermis and the dermis.[12] The strong, resilient epidermis consists of five layers of predominantly dead, but also developing, cells, and functions as a protective shield to the more vulnerable dermis, which contains blood vessels, nerve endings, sweat glands, hair follicles, and connective tissue, and the subcutis, which is a layer of fatty tissue.[13] The aptness of Freud's claim that the ego emerges from our embodied experience is reflected in his idea that our perception-consciousness system functions like a skin. This claim is also foundational to contemporary understandings of surface as revealing of interior workings and thus of primary significance, and yet this surface of perception-consciousness is also layered, like the skin. It is perplexing that Freud himself does not use the metaphor of skin to develop his discussion of the relationship between perception, consciousness, and the unconscious. However, Didier Anzieu, in his career as a psychoanalyst working in the field of dermatology, formulated his own metaphor of the skin ego, which clarifies and extends Freud's concept of the bodily ego.

The Skin Ego

The skin ego is a metaphor that swans over the boundary between British/American and French psychoanalytic schools of thought, and represents this border as porous, rather like its eponymous organ. Anzieu characterizes the division as, on the one side, British/American psychoanalytic theory's empirical approach, which focuses on object-relations and psychogenesis through unconscious happenings in childhood, and, on the other, French psychoanalytic theory's structural approach, which focuses on psychical structures at the expense of an acknowledgment of the importance of experience in shaping structure.[14] It should also be noted that Anzieu is specifically theorizing contra Lacanian psychoanalytic theory and its linguistic turn, which he considers overly grounded in philosophy, the humanities, and social science, at the expense of clinical practice.

Since he privileges imagery and clinical experience over what he characterizes as abstract and formalistic theorizing,[15] Anzieu describes the skin ego as a *metaphor* rather than a fully fleshed-out concept. The skin ego metaphor should be understood in the context of twentieth-century European history which, according to Anzieu, is an epoch typified by a "need to set limits."[16] He observes that over the duration of his practice as a psychoanalyst, the features of his patients' anguish have changed from occupying the territories of Freud's neuroses to occupying borderline (between neuroses and psychoses) and narcissistic states. These states occur more frequently due to a greater cultural need to set limits and boundaries.[17] Linking his metaphor of the skin ego to research in mathematics, astronomy, and biology, which, Anzieu notes, has a preference for taking the interface or membrane as its subject over the infinite and limitless, he delineates his project as the theorization of how psychical envelopes are formed, structured, made pathological, and restored.[18] Anzieu's metaphor of the skin ego is described in two significant passages:

> By Skin Ego, I mean a mental image of which the Ego of the child makes use during the early phases of its development to represent itself as an Ego containing psychical contents, on the basis of its experience of the surface of the body.[19]

> From [its] epidermal and proprioceptive origin, the Ego inherits the dual possibility of establishing barriers (which become mechanisms of psychical defence) and filtering exchanges (with the Id, the Super-Ego and the outside world).[20]

The skin ego exists in the realm of phantasy;[21] like all psychical activity, it is reliant upon a biological foundation (in this case, the skin).[22] Skin is our original communicative interface with the world: "The original form of communication but in reality, and more intensely, in phantasy, is direct, unmediated, from skin to skin."[23] This deep connection between our biological and psychical lives establishes the foundation of sensory experience. According to Anzieu, this "structural primacy" occurs because the skin is an organ that envelops the entire body and also because it is the medium through which we first communicate with the exterior world; therefore, we relate each of our senses to this fundamental sensory experience.[24] To be more precise, the sensory pre-eminence of skin is important not just as a foundation of the senses, but also as a foundation for the reflexivity of our senses.[25] Anzieu elaborates on Freud's discussion of touch as reflexive and the child's experimentation with touching as unique in that the child can apprehend being a touching skin and a touched skin at the same moment.[26] Touching one's self is the precondition of being able to hear one's self talk, see one's self gaze in the mirror, and smell one's own scent (the examples offered by Anzieu).[27] Anzieu traces this discussion about the reflexivity of skin back to Freud's statement in "The Ego and the Id" that the body's surface produces the doubled effect of internal and external sensitivity:[28] as such, the skin is a surface that is both reflexive and doubly perceptive from the interior and exterior. From this reflexivity Anzieu infers that the skin ego consists of two layers, like the epidermis and dermis or the celluloid and waxed paper of the mystic writing-pad, "one turned towards exogenous stimulation, the other towards internal instinctual excitations."[29] While this conclusion connects most obviously to the skin's mediation of the interior and exterior world in cosmetic surgery narratives (as this mediation is reflexive), it also indirectly connects to the contingency of the touch.

The passages that describe Anzieu's skin ego highlight two main characteristics of the metaphor: the skin ego holds the contents of the psyche, and the skin-origin of the ego leads the ego toward its functions as barrier and filter. The skin ego parallels the biological skin's unique abilities to literally hold us together but, unlike an ordinary container, which is rigid, the skin (ego) simultaneously mediates exchange between the interior and exterior of our bodies. As in Freud's discussion of the relationship between consciousness, the ego, and the id, according to Anzieu, the skin ego acts as an intermediary between the inside and the outside: the self distinguishes the psychical ego as its own, and separates this psychical ego from the bodily ego, which is prone to seductive and persecutory influence.[30] What separates the psyche from the body, and in so doing dissolves this separation, is the skin ego: an entity that cannot function without the integration of both. The psychical ego supports a narrative of one's self as a coherent and rational being, and the ego's separation of psychical from bodily ego represents a desire to shunt off the uncontrollable and real effects of the body. The cosmetic surgery patient might seek surgery as a means to counter this uncontrollability, but in so doing is thrown into confrontation with the contingent nature of the body (since surgical results are entirely unpredictable).

The skin ego relies anaclitically on the functions of the skin to determine its own topography: holding the psychical contents together as if a container or sac, acting as an interface between the interior and exterior, and as a communicative surface that can also bear inscription.[31] One of the skin ego's functions is the offering of a "narcissistic envelope" that gives us the fundamental psychical sense of safety that we require in order to interrelate with the world,[32] a response to the differentiation within the ego. Feeling that we belong in our skins, and that our skins belong to us, is tantamount to feeling emotionally and physically protected. This envelope is narcissistic and non-perverse because it requires taking one's own skin/self as loved object in the interests of self-preservation and self regard.[33] The skin ego emerges because the child's experiences of the world are mediated by its body and particularly by its skin (breastfeeding is an exemplar of skin to skin/world contact), and the child thinks about its psyche as contents that are encased within a skin. Likewise, cosmetic surgery tests the skin ego by reaffirming the skin's remarkable capabilities to self-repair, thus mirroring one's psychical ability to hold the self together. The testing of the skin points to the metaphor, in cosmetic surgery, of the skin as a soft clock on which the passage of time is recorded and from which it is effaced, and the boundary of the interior and exterior is rigidified into a fantasized exteriority.

The biological skin is capable of bearing the marks of the exterior world and of others' significations. From the skin's function as a storytelling surface, Anzieu proposes that the skin ego is the foundation and inspiration of thought,[34] and likewise that writing and speech can function like a skin.[35] The poignant affiliation between the skin (ego) and thought is particularly salient in the case of cosmetic surgery, where the cosmetic surgical intervention can be conceptualized as a type of inscription upon the surface of the skin. This inscription may be evident only to the patient, but if we take up seriously this intimate connection between skin and thought, cosmetic surgery is a way of thinking through the skin. When a part of the body becomes a locus of dissatisfaction due to its nonconformance with the self's reading of what the body ought to look like, to declare this a case of bad body image or to claim that this reading is mistaken or overblown is to dishonour and trivialize that dissatisfaction. Or, rather than adopting a definition of "body image" that is common to feminist critique (where body image is understood as an incorrect assessment of one's body influenced by advertising and the media), we can take seriously Paul Schilder's definition of body image as an imagined, yet very real experience. The latter definition is more productive in my considerations of cosmetic surgery because it does not dismiss the fleshiness of our body-thoughts and offers us a framework from which to understand how an intervention into the body can be a productive way to work though psychical dissatisfaction. Further, to understand a dissatisfaction with the body as primarily socially influenced misses the point that the skin is a container, interface, and inscriptive surface for the psychical dissatisfaction and that this dissatisfaction is transposed onto the skin as the bearer of thought and meaning. In this way we can say that the practice of cosmetic surgery transpires on and underneath the skin, and is a thought-negotiation of the boundaries of the skin ego within the consideration of standards of femininity and beauty. These intentional marks of cosmetic surgery are in response and opposition to the unintentional mark of the body, and are a way of negotiating accident, time, and boundaries. Through this line of thought we can see that surface imaginations are not trivial, but central to how identity is formed and lived through the surface of the body.

Contingency

Particularly troubling about the contingent qualities of skin is the fact that the chain of events that leads to a particular manifestation of the skin can be internal or external (or indeed, often confounds the boundary); thus, there is no possibility for protection. Contingency writes itself upon the skin by accident, marking the passage of time and life events in a way that is uncontrollable. The pre-surgical skin is experienced as a contingent organ in cosmetic surgery narratives. What happens to the skin seems to occur by happenstance or accident, or seems dependent on unknown conditions of the future, present, or past. In many of the interview narratives, cosmetic surgery is a way of navigating this contingency, and holds out the promise that surgery can manage the anxiety that arises from the skin's contingency. However, as the interviews demonstrate, cosmetic surgery can only ever partially fulfill this surface imagination-infused promise: the patient and surgeon are unable to assert total control over the cosmetic surgery procedure, for the results are unpredictable. This is a fundamental challenge to the promise made by the surface imagination logic of the photograph, which effects transformation easily and without contingency. In stark contrast to the photographic surface, the skin's surface possesses a frustrating accidental quality as it forms wrinkles, stretch marks, and scars, making it a de-idealized site in the practice of cosmetic surgery.

The Gravity of Age (Tigerlily, lower face, neck, and eye lift)
As you age,
Strange things
happen
to your features.

That really bothered me a lot; every decade another thing.

When my neck started going,
I was sixty.
I remember being very surprised
Because my parents didn't have as much of a turkey neck.

The gravity had set in.

I had this
downward
pull
to
my
face.

I looked miserable, unhappy, cross or sour.

Which did not reflect how I felt in the least.

Thinking about the skin as an object in cosmetic surgery collapses the distinction between the *cutis*, or the skin that is alive, protective, and receptive, and the *pellis*, the skin that is lifeless and subject to textile treatment such as tanning, cutting, and sewing.[36] Connor says that the marking of the skin instantiates the renunciation of skin as a part of the living creature and the objectification of skin into a two-dimensional *pellis*.[37] Cosmetic surgery is always a marking of skin, even in its most non-invasive forms. The mark that cosmetic surgery leaves on the body commemorates the moment that the *cutis* folded into a *pellis*. This figurative death engenders a rebirth of the skin into a condition that manages anxiety through a negation of the contingency of the skin's marks. When I interviewed Tigerlily, she described the contingent and "strange" marks of her skin as a "deterioration or when gravity sets in." The transformation of Tigerlily's skin is not within her control and is instead the result of a gravitational or otherwise mysterious force. Tigerlily described herself as still "energetic," which was in stark contrast to the adjectives that she used to describe her face, such as "miserable," "sour," "cross," and "hideous" because of what she called her "turkey neck" and hooded eyes. She "wanted to reflect to the outside world more of how [she] felt," and in describing her face and neck as parts of a turkey and cloaked in an obscuring skin, she marked these parts as separate from her authentic, interior self. The objectification of her face and neck facilitated an intervention at the level of skin that Tigerlily described as "repulsive" and "frightening" due to the opening up of the skin and unknowability of the results. We can think of this as a response to the objectifying and anxiety-ridden folding together of *cutis* and *pellis* and the accidental quality of all revisions to the skin, even the ones we may choose.

The post-surgical skin has undergone a transformation that writes the skin's vulnerability onto its surface in the form of a bruise, a hole, or a scar. The mark of the surgical intervention corresponds to another of Connor's insights: since one's skin is an object of time, it can only be revised,[38] because the skin's markings are sites through which we experience contingency and law.[39] The skin's marks are frequently experienced as arbitrary and senseless because they do not emerge from our conscious will, as Tigerlily's story attests. Cosmetic surgery is a surface imagination technique for managing the contingency of the skin and the anxieties that arise from its display. Most often, others visually apprehend our skins before they embrace them by the other senses, and we think of the skin as revealing our interiors regardless of our wishes. Tigerlily's story, with her discussion of the effects of lighting and makeup that helped to more accurately reflect her inner self, which was neither "cross" nor "sour," presents this view of the skin. In a peculiar paradox, however, we also strongly adhere to a notion that our skins fail to reveal the entirety of our being: a common saying is that beauty is only skin deep, for example. Cosmetic surgery is a means to conceal time's contingent writing upon the skin,[40] and is a distancing of one's self from accident, decay, and death.

Skin is remarkably vulnerable and yet often an opaque obstacle between the self and the world. The vulnerable obstacle of skin is a site of shame, since it fails to consistently conceal or disclose the interior life and is thus persistently misread culturally.[41] Leah identified stretch marks on her breasts as "the most significant reason" for deciding to obtain a breast reduction and lift. This reason seems incongruous with other more commonsensical reasons for getting a breast reduction, such as back and neck pain, considering large or pendulous breasts aesthetically unappealing, or being fed up with unwanted public hypersexualized and fetishized attention. In fact, having a breast reduction will not do anything about stretch marks, which is something Leah was fully aware of when she went into surgery. She asked her doctor if the reduction surgery would help conceal the stretch marks, and if not, could he "throw some skin on top of there?" The hope expressed in this request is that the surgeon can perform the same alchemy that the photographer can by adding a layer (or filter) over top of the flawed skin to airbrush its contingency.

Leah discussed at length the use of clothing to conceal her stretch marks throughout her history of possessing breasts: "throwing some skin on top of there" would hide the marks in a way analogous to clothing. She did not "need" her breasts because she had no "use" for them. Leah said, "I wasn't worried about [them being] too small, because I was sort of like, honestly, you can take them all, I'm not attached." Like Tigerlily, Leah separated the marks on her breasts from her self as "not-her" due to their accidental quality, conceiving of the self as intentional. Leah described the use of large breasts as purely exhibitory: since she did not show them off, it was unnecessary for her to have them. Since she expressed feeling shame and embarrassment regarding her breasts, the stretch marks operate as a synecdoche for the shame of coming to occupy a highly charged symbol of femininity. Leah's attachment to her breasts was filled with ambivalence about femininity: "I wanted to have the surgery [to] get rid of them *a little bit,* because I really don't need them for anything ... but I still want to, *like I'm still a woman* [and] I still want to be *feminine* and I still want to you know, *have breasts* but I just don't need the full package." Stretch marks are a contingent mark on the skin that remember a time of great physical transformation, and the "full package" of femininity is one of showy surface exhibition (of breasts in particular).

Surprisingly, even though Leah's breast reduction surgery left large and noticeable scars on her breasts, she was completely comfortable with these scars. According to analyst Barrie M. Biven, feeling shame and embarrassment upon one's skin is a strain on one's sense of self-cohesion, and this is often expressed as a desire to escape from, cut, or mutilate the skin as a way to re-establish boundaries and self-cohesion.[42] Often fantasy is a sufficient way of coping with this strain, and Biven explores the everyday projection of one's skin onto living and inanimate objects as a way of negotiating bodily boundaries. The painter's relationship to the canvas is one example of such a projection. The contingently marked and injured skin causes psychic distress not because it represents a biological threat to the organism, but because it disturbs the integrative psychical function of the skin. Connor says that the powerful libidinization of the skin cannot be separated out from a desire for integration through the skin.[43] Given that Leah's happenstance stretch marks concerned her a great deal, while the deliberate scars did not (even though, in all likelihood, they were considerably more pronounced), we might think of Leah's surgery as serving an integrative function. She compared what she calls the "burden" of her breasts and stretch marks to a large "ink stain" on a skirt that her surgery made smaller and less noticeable, making her "happier with [her] body" and her life more "manageable." The stretch marked breasts are the accidental ink stain in Leah's narrative of her body, and cosmetic surgery functions as a stain remover that tries to clean up and control this accident that is visible to everyone on the surface. Leah's surgery allowed her to "look at [her] body and say okay, this is, like, this is what it is now, like things are not really going to change that much anymore." Although it is likely that this statement is not true, and that her body will experience significant change throughout her life, Leah appears to have made herself more comfortable in her own skin through her surgery, and the surgery allows her to put some distance between her present and her past uncontrollable changes.

Tonya's interview narrative is the most starkly contingent story, paralleling the contingency of the skin itself. When Tonya went for a physical in her early twenties, her family doctor found a lump in her breast and she was referred to a specialist. The lump turned out to be benign, but at this appointment the specialist asked Tonya if she had ever considered a breast reduction. This off-the-cuff question turned out to be the spark for a series of appointments that led to Tonya's breast reduction. Tonya had never before considered the possibility of a breast reduction. Her narrative is conceptually structured around unknowingness. Very early in the interview, when Tonya discussed seeing the "boob specialist" who first suggested the breast reduction, she said that she had never even heard of breast reduction, and so she had never considered it. Tonya also said that she had no idea about differences between surgeons and the high variation of skill levels in surgery. When describing her constipation post-surgery, she said that she "never even heard of constipation." The pain she experienced was unfamiliar, a "whole body" pain that was unlike the familiar pain of cuts and burns. The unknown, like the contingent and accidental, is impossible to predict. Tonya tells a surface imagination narrative that envisions a deeper truth beyond the surface (medical procedures beyond the routine physical, layers of surgical skill, interruptions to unthinking digestive function, and deep interior pain). Tonya presented her experience with cosmetic surgery as a journey in which she navigated through unknown surface imagination territory in order to change her detested breasts.

Tonya's narrative is one of lucky accidents that occur as she works through unknown circumstances. While Tonya expressed feeling unconcerned about side effects or possible mishaps, this did not mean that she approached her surgery without any anxiety. For example, she was very concerned that she would be required to remove the barbell in her tongue

piercing prior to her surgery. She was grateful to have her mother present for her surgery because her mother could be relied on to replace the
barbell after the surgery. Tonya commented that she does not "know why,
maybe [she] was just fixating on that, maybe [she] was just projecting all
of this anxiety that I was not allowing myself to have onto my tongue
ring," and that perhaps what she was trying to do was "regain a sense of
self after [her] operation."

Because Tonya's experience with her doctor was so alienating and distanced, it makes sense that she would place such a high value on retaining the tongue piercing after the surgery. Tonya felt the removal of the
barbell as a de-personalization that transformed her body into the generic
body of a breast reduction surgery patient. She felt this acutely in her appointments with the doctor, who made no eye contact and had no time
for her questions. This hole in the tongue's skin might be thought of as
an integrative hole before and after Tonya's surgery. In other words,
Tonya's "fixation" on the barbell is a struggle to make sense of, and gain
some control over, what feels like an unruly bodily experience.

The next contingent skin happening that Tonya discussed at length
was the removal, resizing, and replacement of her nipples during the surgery. Breast reduction surgeries are commonly performed by removing
the nipples and then creating a vertical incision from the nipple that extends into the crease underneath the breast (sometimes referred to as the
"anchor incision" due to its appearance). Tissue is removed from the
breast, the breast is reshaped and lifted, and the incisions are closed. At
the same time, the nipple is cut to a smaller size and then reattached in a
higher position. Tonya was fascinated by this procedure, and describes it
as both "weird" and "awesome," saying that "all [she] could think of
was like [her] nipple just being beside [her] on the, like in a little Petri
dish." What Tonya describes is a fantasy of separating from one's skin,
as a way of experiencing greater closeness and intimacy with the world
and others. Her fascination about the post-surgical nipples combines the
fantasy of escaping the skin, the integrative function of cutting into the
skin, and is a symbol for her of controlling this experience and her body.
As I was packing up after our interview, Tonya told me that she got a tattoo on her chest after the surgery as a "finishing touch." This is entirely
consistent with the trajectory of Tonya's story, which moves from the

contingent and unknown qualities of her skin and the surgery to asserting control over the surgical event that was happening upon her body. The importance of replacing the tongue piercing, the fascination of the removed and restored nipple, and the conclusion of the tattoo are connected together as responses to the accidental and contingent traits of Tonya's surgical narrative.

While Victoria's and Diana's narratives are quite different from those of Tonya, Leah, and Tigerlily, they share a frustration with the skin's obstinacy and refusal to respond to their efforts to change their skins. Victoria explains her skin's contingency through the uncontrollability of biological activity (hormones and reactions to food). Her hopes that what she was experiencing was just a "hormonal thing" set limits on the skin's predictability: eventually, the skin-sky will clear up, so to speak. The primary way that Victoria tried to control her skin was through diet, but eventually she realized that her skin was "very infected" and that she could not control the unruly bacteria on her face. Victoria's solution traded one contingent situation for another. While her acne is uncontrollable and she is not able to predict how it will react to various food, hormonal, and stress situations, the treatment she receives is similarly unpredictable and "depend[ant] on how [her] skin reacts."

Diana, on the other hand, considered the areas in which she had too much fat to be "lumpy," "not a nice texture," and she idealized smoothness of the skin. These lumps compromised the skin's surface, and even if Diana followed a restrictive diet and exercised extensively, this lumpiness would not go away. This was complicated by the reality that Diana was also recovering from an eating disorder and did not want to put that recovery process in jeopardy. The only way that she was able to get rid of this lumpy fat was through starvation and illness, which seemed to disturb her: Diana loved the way her body looked after a two-week kidney infection, but recognized that she could never sustain the smoothness that her skin possessed during illness. Like Victoria, Diana has not found a strategy to successfully control the contingent way her skin looks. Diana and Victoria conceptualized their decisions as a last resort to achieving their goals, something that they would rather not do but nevertheless accept as their final chance to correct the problems that are happening uncontrollably upon and underneath their skins. It is their failure to control the volatile skin that leads them toward cosmetic surgery, rather than thinking of cosmetic surgery as a first choice to remedy a problem that is occurring on the surface of their bodies.

In his discussion of the integrative function of skin, Connor describes two figures, the bodybuilder and the self-lacerator, who share a surprising lineage with the cosmetic surgery patient. The competitive bodybuilder burnishes the skin covering the muscles to a luscious shine in preparation for competition. Connor calls this "skin mirror."[44] This skin mirror is narcissistic, divisional, and embodies the fantasy of an exterior without an interior through the seamlessness and rigidity of its surface. This smooth surface resists the contingency of the skin's marks. When describing someone who has had noticeable cosmetic surgery, the adjective "plastic" is used, but not in the same way as in "plastic surgery." "Plastic surgery" is surgery that has as its aim the reconstruction or alteration of the body, and here "plastic" refers to the capacity to be moulded. The descriptor "plastic" to describe someone's cosmetic surgery outcome instead refers to the hard, often shiny synthetic material, and indicates that the person now appears artificial. The inference here is that the operated upon skin has undergone a hardening or polymerization that undermines the humanity of the soft skin.

Like the bodybuilder, the cosmetic surgery patient might be thought of as sheathed in an idealized psychical exoskeleton that holds the psyche together. Through surgical intervention, the cosmetic surgery patient asserts a control over the contingencies of life and creates an exterior shell that resists the body's insistence on marking one's life in an accidental, haphazard manner. For example, the second degree burning of Victoria's skin through a chemical peel reveals a new skin layer that promises to resist acne and scarring, even if just for a short while. While her hormonal patterns are mysterious and unpredictable, the predictable healing period post-chemical peel is not, and offers control through the skin's dependable ability to heal. Diana's liposuction smoothes out the skin that is lumpy and not a good "texture," and leaves an area that does not bear the marks of the detested, obstinate fat. Her liposuction levels the skin's contingency and its smoothness holds Diana together in her narrative.

The self-lacerator inscribes marks onto the skin that are signs of despoilment. This skin inscription articulates a break in the shining skin mirror, and embraces the contingency of the skin's marks paradoxically through an intentional mark. Although the skin mirror and the skin inscription may appear at first blush to be opposites, Connor says that they share the ideal of an impermeable, smooth surface since the self-lacerator is able to hold the skin together in spite of the damage done to the skin.[45] Both the skin mirror and the skin inscription serve to affirm the skin as a boundary between interior and exterior and as a powerful binding container. The self-lacerator and the cosmetic surgery patient share a desire to re-establish their psychical containers as intact through the intentional breaking through, and reparation of, their skins. Whether it is the bodybuilder's wound inflicted from the inside out or the self-lacerator's wound inflicted from the outside in, the closing up of the chosen wound reaffirms the psychical skin's integrity in spite of its vulnerability, performing an integrative function. For example, while Leah's stretch marks remain exactly the same after her breast reduction, and her scarring is magnified because of the operation, her surgery fashions breasts that belong to her because she has created them. Tonya's narrative is highly invested with the valour of surgery as a means to assert control over the body through the deliberate wounding and healing to effect some sort of change. By making herself vulnerable through permitting the act of incision into her breasts, Tonya asserts her agency.

Time

Gradual and sudden change is marked upon the skin – lastingly and temporarily – through wrinkles, scars, tanning, bruises, and cutting.[46] The slow transformation of our skin over time might one day shock us as we gaze upon a new wrinkle or mole in the mirror, while the healing of a nasty bruise or the fading of a scar may amaze us when one day we can no longer tell where it once was. These physical processes are archaic ways of recognizing the passage of time on our bodies. In my interview conversations, several of the interviewees described the healing time as being like a cocoon or holding tank, a period of time when their bodies recovered from the injuries of their surgeries before they could experience the full results. Cosmetic surgery establishes a second skin, one that marks the patient as psychically resilient. Both Leah and Tonya are highly concerned with the skin's ability to bear marks, particularly stretch marks and post-surgical scarring. Their scars mark a victory over the contingency of the skin and the body, and situate time into a before and an after surgery, like the photograph. Victoria's story of her acne treatments is a bridge between the breast reduction surgeries and the facelifts, because her surgery involves both the creation of a temporary second skin (the crust of the chemical peel) that camouflages acne scarring and also reveals a more perfect second skin underneath.

Next I consider Nicanor's and Tigerlily's facelifts, which established a second skin in a way that could be thought of as a reversal in comparison to Leah's and Tonya's surgeries. For Nicanor and Tigerlily, cosmetic surgery was indeed (as Connor suggests) an attempt to recuperate time through face-lifting surgery since the skin on their faces was showing that too much time had passed in their lives. Their second skin needed to be revealed, rather than created. And finally, I discuss Diana's second skin, which displaces the biological skin and replaces it with a fabric skin (a foundation undergarment). This second fabric skin inscribes a time of indeterminacy and transformation for Diana, a time when she needs the fabric to hold her together until she is able to re-establish her body image and differentiate it from the time prior to her liposuction.

A central contradiction in Leah's narrative is that while she sought surgery in order to address the accidental scarring of her breasts by stretch marks, she was not concerned that the surgery would create new, more prominent scars and would have no effect on the stretch marks. The stretch marks contingently marked her body as feminine in her narrative, and yet the surgical scarring was described as a "non-issue." However, while Leah expressed nonchalance about her surgical scars, she also expressed that they are quite significant to her as a mark that commemorates her refusal of the previous contingent scarring of the stretch marks. These scars form a second intentional skin upon Leah's breasts and inaugurate a new time in her embodied history.

Frankenstein's Bride (Leah, breast reduction and lift)

I looked like Frankenstein's bride first
Because, you know, the stitches are still
Everything's very apparent
The scars are

there.

They are noticeable
I'm not sure how the scars would affect someone else
Who didn't have stretch marks before undergoing a breast reduction
I certainly probably didn't take as good of care of them as I should have.
I was sort of like, who cares?
I was almost giddy.

Leah's account of her recovery and healing period emphasized the extraordinary capacity of the skin to heal. She felt that since she was "already dealing with" scarring from the stretch marks, the potential for scarring was "not going to change [her] life at all." When she first saw her post-surgical body, she described it as "ooh and ahh at the same time,"[47] a simultaneous source of disgust and fascination. She described her body as looking like "Frankenstein's bride" at first since the stitches were very noticeable and "everything's very red and … painful." Frankenstein's bride is a powerful figure of the monstrous feminine, a man-made woman created for a man-made man. Her body is composed of the dead: a past that ought to have been left to the past but instead is forcibly jettisoned into the future as a hybrid human creature. Combining feminine powers of birth and mastery of sewing with masculine desires to surpass death and appropriate birth, Frankenstein's bride is a surgical creation that encapsulates the surgeon-artist's desire to create the body anew and the fantasy of the mutable body held out by cosmetic surgery. In comparing her post-surgical body to the body of Frankenstein's bride, Leah evokes a curious time relation in which the past is unnaturally pushed into the present and future. Her breast reduction refashioned the contingent scarring of stretch marks into the chosen scarring created by the surgeon and consented to by the patient, which is a simultaneous rejection and acceptance of scarring as an embodied process. While the scars are very present for Leah, she views her reconstructed breasts as "almost exactly what I could have wanted, like the best I could have hoped for."

In her reflections on the scarring process, Leah stated, "everything was different, but like the scars are there." The scars left behind from the breast reduction surgery overwrite the stretch mark scars, making it easier for Leah to accept the former scars over the latter. The scar is the mark of time that closes the book on the contingent past and opens up the future. Leah envisions the future of her post-surgical body in a static fashion, stating that it will not change. The scars mark the seams of Leah's second, chosen skin, which she imagines to lack the capriciousness of the first, contingent skin, fixing the body's time into place. They are an important reminder of the surgical event and Leah's decision. Unlike the stretch marks, which she worked very hard to conceal, Leah did very little during the healing process to reduce the appearance of the surgical scars.

Tonya's story of breast reduction is very different from Leah's, as she was quite concerned with the possibility of scarring and did everything possible to minimize the development of visible scar tissue after her surgery. For example, she took turmeric for weeks prior to her surgery and applied creams fastidiously afterward. The only request she remembered having for the surgeon was to look at photographs of people who had undergone a breast reduction, so that she could examine what the scarring looked like. Her scar reduction regimen meant that her scars were "quite good," according to Tonya. She "remember[s] promising [her]self that … after surgery [she] would never be ashamed of [her] scars." And in fact, Tonya goes beyond simply not being ashamed of her scars to proclaiming that she now *likes* her scars. The possible meanings of the scar might explain this turnaround in Tonya's narrative.

When Tonya told me about how she felt after the surgery, she said that she woke up in "a lot of pain," had difficulty walking, found the staples that held together her incisions "huge," and that overall it was "disgusting." She said that she looked like she'd "gone through a Mack truck or something." Tonya described the initial afterward of surgery as agonizing, and she oscillated between describing this pain as originating from the incisions or from the whole body, and totally foreign. Years before her operation, Tonya was in a serious car accident in which she sustained facial injuries. Since she had already seen herself heal to a "normal" condition from a "grotesque" and "horror movie" one, the bruising and swelling post-breast reduction surgery was more manageable. This car accident provided her with evidence of the skin's reparative abilities and gave her hope that her skin would hold her together in the face of grave damage. In spite of being so concerned about scarring after her surgery, Tonya arrived at a conclusion similar to Leah's about her post-surgical scars. Tonya accepted her breasts after her surgery, "even though they were scarred and disgusting and ugly," and embraced her scars as a commemorative mark. The breast reduction surgery tested out the resilience of the skin in a deliberate manner, repeating the satisfaction of the recovery from the car accident's trauma but with an agency that was absent in that past moment. The scars seal Tonya's promise to herself as an inscription into her skin and introduce a new time of power, confidence, and security into her embodied history.

Every Decade Another Thing! (Tigerlily, face and neck lift)
My neck was looking more like a turkey's,
My eyes were starting to get hooded,
You get little pads of fat in the strangest places,
Mostly, this part, the cheeks, had fallen.
Every decade another thing.

Might be a little yellow,
Like bruising goes yellow,
Blue and yellow.
It does heal pretty fast
But your face certainly is disfigured.

The surgery doesn't really make you again a teenager,
But it makes you look rested.
Now did anybody else notice my turkey neck?
I have no idea, but it bothered me.
A lot.

Tigerlily grappled with the gradual effects of time on her face. Like the changes she noticed in her face and neck, her decision to have cosmetic surgery came about slowly: she mulled over the possibility for roughly seventeen years before deciding to go ahead with the face and neck lift. Tigerlily described "coasting" through her fifties on good genes, but the effects of time on her skin bothered her a great deal because, to her, her face did not reflect how she felt. She used the phrase "turkey neck" repeatedly throughout the interview to describe her neck's saggy appearance before surgery. Indeed, the use of this wording throughout our conversation evoked an image of a colourful wattle developing over the years, waving Tigerlily's aging like a flag in the wind. She pinched, tweaked, and pulled the skin under her neck throughout our interview meeting to emphasize that the turkey neck had not been fully remedied by her surgery (even though the surgery had happened almost thirteen years before our interview). While Leah's and Tonya's surgeries created a second scarred skin that promises a less vulnerable future, Tigerlily's and Nicanor's surgeries erased or removed their aging skins to reveal a second, younger skin beneath. The relation to time that Tigerlily's narrative conveyed is that the time of the skin was moving too quickly for her interior clock, and the facelift can be thought of as reversing and arresting time into place.

Nicanor also acquired a second skin in the hope of a second chance for the present and future, although her second chance was bound up with immigration to a new country and hope for occupational promotion. She conceptualized her surgery as a removal of skin and fat, and her second skin did not look dramatically different but rather more "rested" according to others. Nicanor was preoccupied with the relationship between her skin and her past, on the one hand, and what her skin portended for her future, on the other. Her skin is a direct connection to her detested grandmother, as well as the surface onto which her mother projected her own anxieties about femininity and beauty. According to Nicanor, her skin also suggested to others that she was much older than she was. While she acknowledged that sexism in the workplace created this disparity between her chronological age and apparent age, Nicanor still felt that obtaining a facelift would improve her future. Her facelift never appears upon her skin (another difference between Nicanor/Tigerlily and Leah/Tonya[48]), but instead is held within this skin's memory. The alteration of her skin is a return, just as Tigerlily returns to an earlier version of her skin; while this might be conceptualized as a return, it is a return that is effected through the creation of a second, protective skin.

Nicanor recalled talking about scarring with her doctor: it was "sort of [her] concern" that she would develop keloidal scarring because she was Hispanic-American. She said that her "type of olive dark skin tends to heal very ugly." Nicanor further racialized the possibility for scarring by referring to "our type of skin," which added a layer of risk to the surgery that she quickly dismissed as "not my case." It is unclear whether

Nicanor is talking from her perspective or the surgeon's perspective, but these perspectives are quite likely blended. Nicanor connects her skin to a racialized history that could turn up on her face in the form of a scar.[49] This concern with scarring is different from the concerns that Tonya and Leah shared, because in face-lifting surgery scarring is to be avoided completely, whereas in breast reduction surgery it is considered inevitable. Nicanor's surgery detached her current self from her familial past, and her concerns with a particular type of scarring as a racial trait might be related to this desire for detachment. However, Nicanor's conversation with her surgeon about scarring was not the only time she mentioned scarring in our interview meeting. Earlier in the interview, Nicanor discussed the difficulties of having to travel to a Canadian urban centre from a northern Canadian city for the facelift. She explained to her employer that she needed surgery to manage a hard scar left over from a previous eye surgery. This old childhood scar possessed the qualities of the feared keloidal scarring, and referred back to Nicanor's past, but it also provided the necessary proof for Nicanor to leave her job for two weeks to obtain her facelift. While the old facial surgery left a mark, Nicanor wanted to ensure that the second skin of the facelift does not retain marks that can link her face to its past.

Victoria's skin similarly bore unwanted scarring, although her scarring was different from Nicanor's in that it was recent and further blemished by acne. To address this scarring and blemishing, she was in the midst of a long series of chemical peel and laser treatments. There are several types of chemical peels that differ in severity, but they all work on the same principle: by wounding the skin through a chemical burn, the blemished upper layers of the skin are removed to stimulate the growth of new layers of skin. Victoria's chemical peels literally remove false blemished skin by creating a dry crust that peels off over the course of a week to reveal a second, more perfect skin underneath. The chemical peel's creation of a temporary crusty skin that peels off to reveal a more beautiful second skin below affirms Victoria's story that her skin is merely going through an uncharacteristic time but that her real skin is close underneath.

Little Holes (Diana, liposuction on back and abdomen)

I wasn't feeling,

like you're leaking and you're not feeling very social.
You don't really have incisions,
you just have little holes,
So the water kind of leaks out.

I think you're supposed to wear something for the first two weeks, but
you don't have to,
I think the support,
It's like this really thick thing that velcroes around me,
The other option was just to wear
... like, um, like ...
You can get them at department stores.
It's like women's underwear that's all one piece.
Like the bra and panties,
that was much more comfortable.

So long as there's some pressure on the area, I guess.

A common side effect of liposuction is that as the fat and other tissues
redistribute after the operation, a "dip" or a "dent" forms in the skin in
an area where there is not enough fat. The patient must visually monitor
the liposuctioned area closely, and push fat back into the dip if it forms.
Diana was given a waist cincher at her operation that needed to be worn
constantly in order to prevent dips in the skin. It velcroed tightly around
her body but was bulky and uncomfortable underneath clothing, so she
purchased a one-piece women's foundation garment to wear for the two
weeks following her surgery, which was more comfortable. It seemed to
make her feel more secure during the period when fluid was leaking from
the liposuction sites. The kind of foundation garment Diana purchased
is a garment that attaches a bra and panties with stretchy, tight-fitting
fabric, covering the body like a one-piece bathing suit. This is a rather
old-fashioned item of clothing, a skin that reaches back into the past, a
past that Diana herself has not experienced but that kept her intact during a time when her body image had been decimated in her self-image.

The fantasmatic relation between skin and time is a significant force
in cosmetic surgery's fantasy and idealization of the mutable body, for
cosmetic surgery promises to reproduce the reparative miracle of the

skin.[50] As an intervention into the skin, cosmetic surgery leaves behind the mark of time that is incorporated into the skin ego. The surgical intervention establishes a limit or boundary that relies on a temporal element (the before and after). In the psychic time of retroactivity and deferred action, the surgical narrative of the skin connects divergent moments in the chronological history of the skin with the experience of surgery in order to tell the story. Time is a way of organizing random experiences of the skin into language and story, and because the skin's relation to time is contingent, it is a suitable starting point from which to talk about cosmetic surgery. While our bodies bear the marks of time, they also mark time's passage.[51] The intimate affiliation between time and writing that Connor references mimics the intimate affiliation between skin and thought that Anzieu discusses. Connor says that the writing of time on our skins is unintentional, and that the manner in which skin writes time is by effacement.[52] Our bodies live in time, which means that they decay.[53]

Connor's argument that cosmetic surgery is a defence against decay can only travel if we consider surgeries that aim to make the patient appear younger. Certainly many cosmetic surgeries could be considered as anxious defences against aging and decay, but how might we think about surgeries such as breast reduction and liposuction, which can possibly transform the body into a previously unknown (or known only to the mind) morphology? What is their relation to time? The incisions from these surgeries perform the feat of sundering the skin only to seal it back together, but their relation to time is to mark a before and an after, rather than a return to a fantasmatic past. The facelift attempts to transform the after of the face (aging) and reverse it into the before, and this operation can be performed repeatedly; the breast reduction, on the other hand, alters the skin of the breast in a way that will be marked for the lifetime of the skin. If the skin can be thought of as a "soft clock," as Connor suggests, that can wind time backward after it has been injured, it might also be thought of as a calendar upon which we commemorate a specific moment in time. The scar is this commemorative mark, although if we are to take the skin ego seriously, the scar is not *merely* a commemorative mark since the perforation and healing of the skin can function psychically as an experiment with the skin ego's boundaries. Through memory and affect the skin ego holds on to the experience of surgery and keeps it

close, like the scar. Connor says that the scar is an "arrested scab" because unlike the scab, the scar remains.[54] The scab is an ambiguous entity, one that is neither still an injury nor yet a scar, perpetuating and
transforming the injury into something else: it is "a visual compromise
between lesion and healing."[55] If the pleasure of the scab is the "pleasure
of an averted threat,"[56] the pleasure of the scar is the pleasure of survival
– the pleasure of the second skin. The pleasure of the scar is the enjoyment of the despoiled body and its decay, and in cosmetic surgery the scar
can be celebrated rather than taken as a failure or unhappy ending (as
Connor's understanding of cosmetic surgery might suggest). The creation
of a second skin re-establishes security after the violence of the operation
and holds the body together as an object of time. The scar is also an in-
determinate space between the interior and exterior of the body, a hardening that replaces the skin in the place of the wound.[57]

Interior/Exterior

There is a prevalent belief that the skin reveals our interior life: if an individual is happy, well fed and exercised, and has a clear conscience, the
myth holds that their skin will be unblemished. The ideal of the unblemished skin is coupled with the racist idealization of white skins, where the
unblemished beautiful skin is described using metaphors of whiteness and
light such as "bright," "clear," or "translucent." In cosmetic surgery narratives, the pervasive statement that the patient feels as though her exterior body does not match the way she feels about herself inside is used to
explain the motivations for having surgery. This explanation can be used
to describe surgeries that target signs of aging such as wrinkles and sagging, but it can also be used to explain someone feeling that parts of her
body appear different from how she herself feels.

Tigerlily and Nicanor were both concerned about appearing older
than they were, and appearing older than the age they felt. Growing, and
particularly appearing, older is perceived as a tragedy for women in North
American popular culture, and there is an enormous cosmetics industry
that exists to address these problems. Tigerlily was surprised to begin a
love affair at the age of sixty-five, something she thought would never
happen after the death of her husband. While Tigerlily discussed her new
partner as not a factor in her decision to have surgery, one can imagine

that falling in love is nevertheless a transformative experience that calls to mind all previous instances of falling in love. Tigerlily said that her sagging facial and neck skin made her appear to be "miserable" and "unhappy," which "bothered" her a lot. She felt young (and, as she says, happy because of her new partner), but when she looked at herself she saw instead a "witch." She explained her motivations for undergoing a face, neck, and eye lift in what is a typical manner for these surgeries: the interior and exterior do not match up. On the other hand, Nicanor did not describe her surgery in the same way because she was less concerned about what she thought of her appearance and more concerned about what her appearance meant to other people. Her skin betrayed her too, but she framed this betrayal as having economic rather than social consequences. After she had her face, neck, and eye lift, a friend told her that her face and bones had "more definition" because the skin was stretched more tautly across her facial structure. The stretching of her skin made her look more "rested," according to Nicanor, again raising the notion that the exterior of the skin reflects one's true inner being.

One of Diana's qualms with her skin prior to her liposuction was that the problematic fat on her back and abdomen was not "a nice texture," which she associated with not being "fit" or "in good shape." Diana provided a surface explanation here; there are no psychological or other motivations given, and perhaps because of her eating disorder, she avoided mentioning other motivations in order to avoid pathologizing her own decision. One of her hopes was that this texture would improve after surgery, yet she repeated that there "has to be more" to her hopes and expectations of the surgery. Being "fit" and "in good shape" are ambiguous, and Diana seems to define these terms on a visual, surface basis even though they refer to overall health rather than appearance. These are qualities that are connected to the skin in their ambiguity. What Diana ostensibly struggled with was the lack of a coherent explanation intelligible by popular discourses of cosmetic surgery, which negate the importance of the surface while reifying it. So while psychological explanations are quite effective in justifying cosmetic surgery and explaining motivations according to interior emotions, the outcomes of the surgery show up on the exterior of the body. Diana's story lines up both the explanation and the outcome onto the exterior of the body, which made her feel like there "has to be more" to her hopes and expectations of the surgery. She grasped at straws, explaining that perhaps she hoped to be more comfortable being naked with other people, which would therefore improve her relationships. This is linked with the mainstream medical treatment of eating disorders, which focuses on how the person with an eating disorder misinterprets what her body looks like and does not see it as it "really" appears. Treatment focuses on building up the interior of the body to be better equipped to cope with one's unrealistic perceptions (and thus, over time, create new "realistic" perceptions of the body's appearance). Instead, Diana worked through her problem on the body's surface, an approach that she saw as "unhealthy" and problematic. Diana's narrative challenges her identity as someone recovering from an eating disorder, because she is deliberately trying to remedy her body image issues through changing the body, rather than her perception – behaviour that is unacceptable according to mainstream treatments for eating disorders. It is difficult to discern whether Diana was telling me about the ways that her surgery might be thought of as an "unhealthy" decision (according to mainstream treatments of eating disorders) because she was struggling with her decision herself, or if she felt that it was responsible to acknowledge her decision in this manner as a feminist and person who was in recovery. To put it another way, Diana was troubled that she was addressing her negative feelings about her body on the surface and according to surface imagination logic that the exterior is more important and can change the interior.

Tonya's story also deviated from more culturally acceptable psychological explanations for cosmetic surgeries. While Tonya expressed a loathing for her breasts, her story was based more on a series of contingent events that led up to her discovery of breast reduction as an option. Tonya hated her breasts prior to her reduction, saying that they "were terrible," that men liked them but that she saw them as a "barrier" or "pain in the ass," and that she did not like the way they looked or felt. She was enthusiastic about having a breast reduction. Tonya said that she was flat-chested when she was young, and that she began menstruating relatively late in comparison to her friends and classmates, at the age of fourteen. Her breasts took her by surprise, as they developed very quickly and became quite big. Interestingly, she switched from initially saying that her breasts were so big, to saying that they were not *that* big, to a more tempered response: "in my head ... they just *felt* [like] these huge monstrosities." I understood this statement as a nod to psychological explanations for cosmetic surgery and acknowledgment that the psychical experience of the body matters just as much as the so-called physical experience of the body.

After her breast reduction surgery Tonya felt more confident, which she linked to being more comfortable having sex with the lights on. She experimented with "different kinds of sexuality" because her surgery freed her sexually: "This is great, I can get naked, I can have sex, it was like a lot more exploratory, which was really good." She did not discuss her surgery with others immediately after she had it, not because she felt any shame or embarrassment but because she described herself as a "private person" who "didn't really talk anything about emotions, so it, it made sense that [she] wouldn't really talk about [her] boob job either." Also at this point in the interview, she described her wardrobe as consisting primarily of baggy men's clothing, because she wanted to hide her breasts and not draw attention to them. A few years after the surgery, however, she described herself as now an "open book" who has spoken to several women about her breast reduction surgery. She is also wearing more fitted men's clothing that does not hide her body. Since Tonya linked her clothing with her general levels of self-confidence and comfort with discussing emotions, as well as with nudity, I think this is one of the ways that Tonya negotiated the relationship between the interior and exterior of her body through the skin. Prior to the surgery, Tonya was uncomfortable with being naked (particularly in the light), wore concealing clothing, and was "private." After her breast reduction, Tonya enjoyed being naked and wore clothing that fitted her and revealed her body. The surgery was a catalyst for Tonya to express her interior life more openly on the surface. The more fitted clothing resembles the skin that Tonya is more at ease showing to others when naked, which is also akin to her more free expression of her emotional life to others.

Tonya also expressed the relationship between her interior and exterior life through her skin using the metaphor of the cut. Unlike the scar or the scab, the cut is the immediate remnant of the wound, more vulnerable to letting the interior contents out and to allowing the exterior environment in. Cutting in Tonya's interview narrative refers to the surgical procedure and incisions but also to the psychical/physical removal of her breasts. One consequence of the repetition of the cut in this interview is that Tonya frequently describes her breasts as being in fragments.

About the appointment that she had with the person she dubs the "boob specialist," Tonya said, "When she suggested cutting them off, it was like, get rid of them!" She met the idea of breast reduction with enthusiasm as a result, and her process happened very quickly. The "boob specialist" also told Tonya that they remove the nipple during the operation, and move "chunks" around in order to accomplish the reduction.

She found the process of removing the nipples during the surgery to be particularly fascinating. She asked the nurse where the nipple went during the surgery (in a little dish), and said that they put it back on when they were "sewing you back up." She also asked if they cut the nipple smaller so that it seems more proportionate to the smaller breast (they do). Finally, Tonya talked about being in women's studies classrooms and discussing female genital cutting, and insinuated that she felt hypocritical about talking about this subject because "I just cut my tits open because I didn't really like them." As these examples demonstrate, Tonya emphasized the physical removal of skin, fat, and tissue. This prospect was exhilarating for Tonya, who could not wait to have surgery once the process got started. She fragmented her breasts into pieces that can be cut up, cut into, or cut off. If we consider this alongside Tonya's slow increase of self-confidence, the cut of the exterior scalpel that breaches the barrier of the breasts' skin to excavate tissue and fat also opens Tonya up psychically. After her surgery, she is able to experiment more with the interplay between concealment and exposure, both through clothing and through emotions and storytelling.

Everything Shows (Victoria, chemical peels and laser treatments)

In my early twenties about two three years ago, my skin like exploded, is how I describe it.

I've had a series of facial treatments for acne.
To clear skin.

I know a lot of people don't think it's associated with diet,
but for me,
I think my type of acne is,
very closely associated with what I eat, yeah,

so,
I really have to be careful about how much fried food and how much
like junk food, like chocolate ...

I felt like when people met me they would say,
oh,
She's a pretty girl,
but
If only she had clear skin, it would be better.

I'm a big believer that everything shows. Like your emotional,
as well as your physical,
Well-being will show through on your face.

Like even if you're not prone to acne.
In your complexion,
Everything shows on the outside.

I'm very health-conscious naturally.
I didn't want,
like you know,
like I put the time into you know, eating right
and going to the gym
and all that kind of stuff.

I didn't want people to look at me
you know, judge me.

Victoria's interview narrative is very invested in the notion that the
skin will expose one's interiority. Unlike Tonya, who maintained that the
skin could conceal or contain the interior life (even if that may happen
through a clothing prosthesis), Victoria insisted that the skin would show
all eventually (even though this contradicts her experience). Victoria had
a heavy investment in the truth-telling capacities of the skin, even though
her own skin deceives the world. While Victoria follows a restrictive diet
regimen, exercises regularly, and maintains a labour-intensive skin care
routine at home, she still gets acne. She is a "big believer that everything

shows," which she further explains as meaning that "your emotional, as well as your physical well-being will show through on your face … in your complexion, and in your eyes, everything shows on the outside." Victoria feels that her acne is unfair and worries that it signals to others that she pigs out on junk food frequently and does not "take care" of herself. Like Diana, Victoria's individual efforts did not alleviate her problem, so she turned to a surface solution to the inaccurate depiction of her interior upon her skin.

Victoria is the only interviewee whose interventions do not puncture the skin's surface. Victoria's actions can be understood as a last resort to manage the exterior of her body, which does not cooperate with the interior and instead presents a misleading story to others. We can understand Victoria's decision to undergo multiple procedures on her skin as directly related to her belief that "everything shows." In Victoria's narrative, the skin is a truth-telling organ that speaks the interior of the body to the world, and she experiences her skin as betraying her by telling lies through its acne. The technicians assist her in delving deeper into her skin to find the truth. The paradox of skin is that while Victoria's belief in the skin's ability to reflect our interior lives to the exterior world is quite common, so is the counter-belief that the skin deceives others and does not express much at all to the exterior world. Victoria's story is a merger between these understandings of skin and beauty, for she insists that it is possible to see one's health upon the skin, and yet her way of treating her own skin's transgressions is through the method of travelling skin deep via laser or acid.

Claudia Benthien's central argument in *Skin: On the Cultural Border between Self and the World* is that the skin is an increasingly unyielding boundary, even though medical science has infiltrated the interior of the body through the skin.[58] One of the current major trends in cosmetic surgery involves delving deeper beneath the skin, and an example of this is the manipulation of the superficial muscular aponeurotic system (SMAS) of the face to achieve a more effective facelift. The other current major trend in cosmetic surgery travels in the opposite direction, with surface treatments that avoid cutting into the skin's boundary, such as the wide variety of injected substances (for example, Botox, Restylane, and collagen), chemical peels, and laser resurfacing. We can understand both trends as responses to Benthien's argument, in that the former attempts to breach the impenetrable boundary of the skin to effect change and the latter seeks to maintain the limits of that boundary. The interior and exterior of the body are held as separate entities, and these two trends in cosmetic surgery parallel two approaches Benthien identifies in idiomatic expressions about skin. First, there are expressions that represent the skin as protective, keeping the self inside and shielding the authentic person from the exterior world. The second class of expressions takes the skin as a synecdochial organ for the whole body and subject, whereby one's authenticity cannot be hidden because it is there for all to see.

Benthien argues that more contemporary expressions and representations of the skin take the position that the skin is a protective shell, but not the whole person. However, as my interview narratives demonstrate, the friction between these two understandings of skin is very much alive and present, and the fantasy held by surface imaginings of the body and culture fuse these two understandings together. Changing one's protective shell can indeed alter the whole person, inside and out. All the narratives I have outlined in this section struggle with these tensions between interior and exterior, and affect and appearance. Nicanor, Tigerlily, and Victoria work through the difficulties that emerge from the incongruity between how the skin appears to the exterior world and the interior of the body, whether that inconsistency is related to one's age or one's health. Diana and Tonya face the complications of explaining their surgeries within a context that privileges the interior life as more authentic, given that their surgeries attempt to change the self by changing the skin's surface. These tensions do not correspond to a specific mode or trend of surgery; Victoria and Diana narrate their experiences of interior and exterior differently, and yet they both have surgeries that aim to leave no permanent mark on the skin. Likewise, Nicanor, Tigerlily, and Tonya all have surgeries that are comparatively physically invasive and leave marks that are to be camouflaged or are inevitable.

In his book *Second Skins: The Body Narratives of Transsexuality*, Jay Prosser asks, "If the skin is a mask, where is the self in relation to the body's surface? Deeper than the skin (underneath the mask)? Or not 'in' the flesh at all?"[59] These questions take the position outlined above that the skin is a shield, protecting the interior self from the exterior world. Benthien argues that an earlier understanding of the body as a house has been replaced over the course of the past two centuries by the idea of the body as dress.⁶⁰ The most significant difference between these two conceptions of the body (skin) that I identify in Benthien's discussion is that the dress is a permeable site of exchange, which certainly corresponds to contemporary surface imagination ideas about the skin. Rather than understanding the window-orifices to be the locations of exchange, the entire surface possesses this capability. The conceptualization of skin in cosmetic surgery is a hybrid of the dress and the house. Benthien identifies five implications of understanding the body as a house whose emptiness is filled by the subject: it is possible to leave or alter the fixed skin; the orifices of the skin can be opened and closed to sensation; the skin is impenetrable; the subject inside the skin is not assimilable to its outside environment; and the skin mediates between the public and private (intimacy is defined as entering the skin through its orifices).⁶¹

Blum describes one interview she conducted with a surgeon who was a proponent of face-lifts at a young age, and he explained his position with recourse to the metaphor of the skin-house: "'Now, if you can argue that age twenty-five is maturity and you had exactly the right amount of skin coming from the brow down to the first fold and exactly the right amount of skin coming to the eyelashes ... and that was normal, then is it normal to allow time to change it, so that the skin begins to slide down over the jaws and the bags begin to show? Well, that's not the way it was when it was twenty-five, anymore than when I painted my house it was natural for me to let it gradually deteriorate. I keep it up – repair and maintenance.'"⁶² Blum remarks that this surgeon uses a specifically middle-class morality to explain his (somewhat) controversial opinion that people ought to consider face-lifting surgery as early as their late twenties. However, his analogy between the skin of the face and the paint on the house is completely compatible with Benthien's description of the body/skin as house, as well as Prosser's questioning about the skin as mask, because they are all linked through surface imagination fantasies that the outside creates and projects the inside back out into the world. In this formulation, the delineation between interior and exterior is blurred because the body is conceptualized as all exteriority. Setting aside the surgeon's assumptions about the twenty-five-year-old face as "normal," he reconfigures a more common understanding that having a facelift in one's twenties is scandalous and unnecessary by recourse to the skin as a house. Recognizing the skin as a house is an important means to explain cosmetic surgery in a manner harmonious with middle-class ideals of respectability through the upkeep and repair of one's property; discourses of home renovations and cosmetic surgery collide in this surgeon's explanation, revealing a shared surface imagination logic to both.

Prosser, in *Second Skins*, attempts to challenge the de-materialization of the transsexual body by queer and feminist theory by rooting his analysis in the so-called physical experience of the body and transition.[63] Benthien's discussion of the contemporary conceptualization of the body/skin as dress is useful and relevant here. Prosser argues that the feeling that one is trapped in their skin or that one possesses the wrong skin is common in transsexual narratives because that *is* what transsexuality feels like.[64] Part of the tragedy of conceiving the skin as dress is that we are resigned to wearing it forever. The skin as house metaphor marks the subject as separate from others through walls and barriers, whereas the skin as dress metaphor marks the subject as separate from others through individuality and expression of identity through appearance. Both metaphors hold pure exteriority as an ideal to be achieved. Prosser remarks that feeling as though one is in the wrong body constitutes a failure to own one's skin or feel it to be one's own.[65] As the interview narratives demonstrate, this is a common thread in explanations of why one might have cosmetic surgery. This statement keeps the interior and exterior of the body separate, and marks the skin as the limit between the inside and outside.

However, if Prosser's statement is pushed a little further, it comes closer to describing the significance of skin in cosmetic surgery narratives. To feel trapped in a mistaken body means to fail to own one's skin, but since the skin itself *is* the body in a surface imagination culture, the mistaken body and the unfamiliar or distant skin are the same thing. The skin in cosmetic surgery narratives (and transsexual narratives in Prosser) collapses together the interior and the exterior into a surface that privileges the exterior. For example, a culture that does not define identity according to the appearance of its surfaces might instantiate a system of re-naming or re-telling body parts, so that *language* rather than *image* would be used to manage the discomfort of being in the wrong skin. As Anzieu argues, feeling as though one has a skin that belongs to them and that can be used for sensory experience is the same thing as being one's self.[66] Prosser understands this to mean that assuming a subjectivity means to not just have a skin, but to have a sense of ownership of one's skin as well as a psychic investment in one's skin.[67] Cosmetic and sex reassign-ment surgery can be thus thought of as a means to own one's skin by accepting the misfortune of wearing the same skin-dress day after day through tailoring it in a way that makes it one's own.[68]

Citing the field of psychodermatology, Prosser remarks that the skin is a "psychic/somatic interface" that is sensitive to external psychical stress, and that, conversely, to have a skin disorder itself is stressful.[69] What occurs here is that one's psychic life transforms the body itself: as Prosser notes, this is an exteriorization of something that is thought of as purely internal. Prosser is talking about the body image, and here intro-duces a different way of thinking about body image from the feminist definition of a false notion of what one's body "really" looks like, and Schilder's definition of a psychical representation of one's body that is no less authentic due to its status as a mental image. Through his use of Anzieu's metaphor of the skin ego, Prosser conjures up body image as a psychical representation of the body capable of effecting physical change. Anzieu states that the imagined or literal mutilating of the skin is a "dra-matic attempt ... to maintain the boundaries of the body Ego and to re-establish a sense of being intact and self-cohesive."[70] While it is rather difficult to separate the word "mutilate" from its moralistic connotations, if we consider "mutilation" to refer to a significant injury to the body or part of the body, cosmetic surgery can indeed be thought of as a mutila-tion of the skin that confirms one's skin as one's own. This is a boundary negotiation that occurs at the level of skin as a location that is neither in-terior nor exterior, nor both, but instead is a hybrid location through which we experience ourselves as separate and connected to the world.

A Speculative Digression on Interiors/Exteriors and Sex Reassignment Surgeries

Frequently, I am asked to comment on the connection between "cosmetic surgeries" and "sex reassignment surgeries" (SRS), which is a good ques-tion, yet one that perplexes me. The truth is, I have little to say about the connection and often reply with something like, "Both have everything to do about gender." This is not a dismissal, but simply an observation that while the practices share an intense interest in gender presentation, the connection between SRS and cosmetic surgery is not self-evident to me, nor is it one taken up extensively by trans studies scholars or by activists advocating for access to SRS. There are, of course, good reasons for this, reasons that are connected to the enduring division between reconstructive and cosmetic surgeries. Conceptualizing SRS as reconstructive or otherwise different types of surgeries from cosmetic surgeries is a strategic move that is often necessary to obtain or advocate for access to SRS. Further, SRS *is* fundamentally different from cosmetic and even reconstructive surgeries since there are levels of institutional surveillance and gatekeeping that the patient seeking a cosmetic or reconstructive surgery does not have to face.[71]

The example of breast augmentation in the Canadian context is particularly illustrative here, and I will focus on Ontario specifically since this is the location within which I conducted my interviews. A non-transsexual woman seeking breast augmentation for cosmetic purposes in Ontario does not need a referral from a family doctor in order to make an appointment with a cosmetic surgeon. At her consultation appointment, she must demonstrate to a cosmetic surgeon that her wish to receive implants is self-motivated and mentally healthy, and not driven by an underlying psychological issue or the result of an external pressure.[72] Her breast augmentation will not be covered by provincial health insurance, and so she will pay for it herself.

A non-transsexual woman who undergoes a unilateral or bilateral mastectomy will be offered breast augmentation as an option to reconstruct her breast(s); she will not need to undergo the same psychological screening as the patient seeking implants for cosmetic reasons, since it is an underlying assumption that this surgery will be psychologically positive. Her breast augmentation will be covered by provincial health insurance.[73]

Finally, a transsexual woman who wishes to obtain breast augmentation can make an appointment with a cosmetic surgeon without a referral from her family doctor, since this surgery will not be covered by provincial health insurance.[74] However, she faces a number of barriers that a non-transsexual woman seeking implants for cosmetic reasons does not. She will need to demonstrate to the cosmetic surgeon not only that she is psychologically sound and self-motivated, but also that she has lived as a woman for at least one year (also called "real life experience") and she must provide two letters supporting her decision to obtain breast augmentation. The first letter must be from a psychologist or psychiatrist, and must diagnose the patient with Gender Identity Disorder/Gender Dysphoria; the second letter must be from a mental health professional who has attained at least a master's level education and has specialized training in the fields of sexuality and gender "disorders." Thus, while a non-transsexual woman seeking breast augmentation must receive the assent of only one gatekeeper (the cosmetic surgeon), the transsexual woman must receive the assent of three gatekeepers (the cosmetic surgeon and two mental health professionals). In this example of just one surgical operation, there are multiple differences between the processes and experiences of women, depending on their reasons for seeking breast augmentation and the meaning of their decision within their societal and cultural contexts.

This is not to say, however, that there are no connections between cosmetic surgeries and sex reassignment surgeries. In this speculation, I wish to situate the question within the context of surface imagination through the shared narrative of the "wrong body." As I discussed in the previous section, I am compelled by the work of Prosser on transsexual autobiographies, in which he considers the body and narrative to be intermeshed. Whether we have cosmetic surgery or not, or whether we are transsexual or not, narrative is a fundamental way that we all establish an intimacy with or estrangement from our own bodies. The narrative of being in the wrong body has proved to be very powerful and resonant across a range of embodied experiences, including individuals who seek cosmetic surgery, transsexual individuals who seek SRS, and transabled individuals who seek a physical impairment or disability.[75] As Prosser argues, and Nikki Sullivan underlines, the narrative of being in the wrong body is not simply a rhetorical strategy, but one that is viscerally experienced and in fact *produces* an experience.[76] Within the Western understanding of the body as one's individual property, as well as the assumption that bodily integrity is critical to the welfare of an individual,[77] surgery becomes a technique that offers access to the right body, which means to truly own the body and inhabit it.

Sullivan explains, however, that this narrative is not as versatile or strategic as it may seem. She locates the narrative of the wrong body as emerging from early sexological discourses of inversion, as well as early to mid-twentieth century treatments of homosexuality. She notes that this narrative was assimilable to biological theories of sexuality and that early sex reassignment surgeries were performed not to change sex but to treat homosexuality (and were justified on that basis).[78] Early SRS endeavoured to produce a new body surface not in order to alleviate the suffering of trans-identified individuals, but to visually transform a sick homosexual man into a healthy heterosexual woman so the individual's sexual practices could better conform to the social body.[79] Although this early treatment is clearly pathologizing and conflates sexuality and gender, it set the stage for contemporary mainstream understandings of SRS, based on the narrative of the wrong body. In a parallel fashion, the cosmetic surgery patient also narrates her experience of embodiment as wrong in relation to a mental image of the body, and this has been a successful strategy within the cosmetic surgery industry.

In sharp contrast, the narrative of the wrong body has not been a successful strategy to explain the embodied experiences of transabled people because, unlike the pre-surgical bodies of transsexual and cosmetic surgery patients, the wrong body of the transabled person is codified as a normal body. Sullivan's analysis is useful, since it highlights how the wrong body narrative is inextricable from the notion of "wrong embodiment" (meaning pathological or abnormal embodiment), and has become the *only* intelligible way to narrativize the ambiguity of embodiment. The wrong body narrative relies on a pathologization of difference, a split between the mind/body, an idealization of wholeness, and an ahistorical and absolute notion of somatic wrongness.[80] Referring to Susan Stryker's work, Sullivan comments that while the wrong body narrative has been successful in obtaining positive outcomes, it also forecloses an analysis of the institutional and systemic relations that make this narrative intelligible and renders others unintelligible, such as transability, queer genders, or cosmetic surgeries to obtain outcomes beyond normative body ideals.[81]

Implicit within the wrong body narrative is a surface imagination tension. The surface of the body is wrong when it does not reflect the interior image of the body, a position that privileges the mind as true over the body as false. This is typically the wrong body position that is used by both pre-surgical cosmetic and sex reassignment surgery patients, in order to justify surgery to others. Yet at the same time, a change to the body's surface to make it "feel right" is understood as so influential that improving the patient's healthy interior life is dependent upon that surface transformation, a position which then privileges the body as the true representative of self. This is the wrong body position that is more commonly expressed post-surgery, which narrates the surface transformation as a catalyst for positive life changes.

What is codified as the wrong or the right body surface in relation to the mental image of the body is not a neutral process; rather, the generally unsuccessful use of the wrong body narrative by transabled people demonstrates that in order for this narrative to be intelligible, the mental image must conform to ideals and norms, and the body surface must fail to conform. In her analysis of normalization in self-transformative practices like transsexuality, dieting, and cosmetic surgery, Cressida Heyes is concerned with this tension between the interior/exterior and its relation to norms and ideals. She notes that the "languages of authenticity and perfectibility" are central to resolving the conflict that exists between interior/exterior.[82] Heyes argues that what is common across all three practices is "the cultivation of a body oriented toward an endpoint."[83] I would add that this endpoint is one that fixes the body through a surface imagination fantasy of the skin as photogenic; that is to say, a fantasy that the body's surface has been altered to become a museological object that represents an authentic interior self. Thus, just as non-trans women must negotiate ideals and norms of femininity when seeking out cosmetic surgeries, so too do these image codes of feminine appearance structure – and potentially limit – the available outcomes for trans women when seeking out sex reassignment surgeries.[84]

None of my interviewees self-identified as transsexual,[85] and while I corresponded with several potential interviewees who underwent various cosmetic surgeries not represented in the narratives in this book, none of them situated their surgeries within the domain of SRS either. The present digression should be read with this in mind, as a *speculation* on what connections exist between the experiences of cosmetic surgery and SRS patients through the concept of surface imagination, but a speculation that exists in the absence of qualitative interview information. I wish to conclude this speculation by proposing that because the visual presentation of the body to others is important to both the cosmetic surgery and the SRS patient, it is likely that individuals who obtain sex reassignment surgeries negotiate a similar compromise between surface imagination expectations (structured by the limitless photograph) and surgical outcomes (structured by the limit of the skin).

For example, in her case study on the importance of being attentive to relational practices of looking with a trans patient in a psychoanalytic psychotherapy setting, Alessandra Lemma proposes that *being seen* is central to experiences of being transsexual.[86] These experiences of *being seen* are organized around an "'incongruity' ... between the given body and the body ... identified as [the] 'true' physical home," and this gap is difficult to communicate and negotiate with others.[87] As Lemma reminds us, Donald Winnicott argues that many individuals "take for granted the lodgment of the psyche in the body and ... forget that this again is an achievement."[88] In her work with transsexual patients, Lemma observes that there is a search for a "dwelling for the self" in the individual's body but also within the mind of an other who could gently hold this experience of incongruity.[89] Accomplishing a "lodgment" of the psyche in the body through the self and others is, of course, not a challenge or accomplishment that is faced by transsexual people alone – every one of us must struggle to negotiate the incongruous experience of being seen by others, of being recognized and misrecognized. Something that cosmetic surgeries and SRS promise to patients is a new body surface that will more accurately reflect the "true" body/self.

Lemma's comments on the psychical effects of sex reassignment surgeries resonate with the narratives of cosmetic surgery discussed in this book. She states that surgery undoubtedly improves the quality of life for transsexual individuals, and in many cases "may be the only way to live."[90] This experience of urgency and post-surgical improvement of quality of life is also expressed by many cosmetic surgery recipients, including my interviewees. However, Ms A (the patient whom Lemma's case study is based upon) encounters a number of complications following SRS, including dissatisfaction with her surgical results, depression, and an experience of intense emotional pain regarding old photographs of herself and her wish to rip them up. Lemma interprets these complications as the "decimation of a fantasy that SRS would take away the pain so concretely located in her body,"[91] and arising from the impossibility of bypassing one's embodied history (a loss) through a surgical intervention.[92] While Ms A changes the surface of her body, this action does not accomplish all the psychical aims she hoped for; after her SRS, she must continue the difficult psychical work of dwelling comfortably in her body. Rather than an endpoint, surgery is often a step on the path to *becoming* a body of one's own. I would argue that this fantasy – that SRS *or* cosmetic surgeries alone can excise psychical pain from the body and transform it into a home – is a surface imagination fantasy, where patients experience psychical and somatic complications as necessary compromises on the path to achieving what Winnicott terms the "psyche indwelling in the soma."[93] Underlining this fantasy is the tension between the interior and exterior of the body, which is experienced particularly through the limit of the skin.

Conclusion

Throughout this discussion, I have explored the manifold topography of skin in cosmetic surgery beginning from the metaphor of the archipelago. Akin to the archipelago's chain of islands fluidly connected and divided from each other by the sea, the skin's psychical and somatic experiences and memories occur in ways that are attached and separated by cultural fluctuations. The skin narratives isolate the skin as the de-idealized surface of cosmetic surgery, and highlight how the skin is the medium within which relations of contingency, interiority/exteriority, and time are rehearsed and played out. Contingency means not knowing what will happen in the skin's history, or what effects the skin's markings will have on the subject in relation to the world. One's sense of interiority and exteriority in conversation with the skin produces a sense that the contingent is exterior and strikes one's interiority through the mark. These thematic understandings of skin lead us to wonder what effect cosmetic surgery might have on one's psychic experience of the skin, and what the incising of the skin does structurally.

Renata Salecl is concerned with how we might theorize the coincidence of a range of contemporary body cutting practices in diverse geographical locations that purport a "return" to traditional body modification practices, such as clitoridectomy in the global South and piercing and tattooing (body art) in the global North. She identifies a common (racist) misunderstanding of clitoridectomy as a return to pre-modern, traditional practices of initiation; however, Salecl argues that contemporary practices of clitoridectomy ought to be considered as postmodern body modification practices.[94] Salecl suggests that we instead consider the contemporary practices of clitoridectomy and piercing as culturally different ways of dealing with the impasses and paradoxes of postmodern societies.[95] This positions distinct contemporary cutting practices like clitoridectomy, piercing, and tattooing not as a *return*, but rather a *reinterpretation* of rites of passage that emerge out of specific postmodern cultural contexts. Salecl fashions her argument around the different ways that contemporary subjects position themselves in relation to the Symbolic structure. While the cultural and geographical contexts are varied, Salecl argues that there is a common thread: namely, the cut to the body is a postmodern way of dealing with the absence of the big (Symbolic) Other of Lacanian theory.

In Lacanian psychoanalytic theory, our psychical experience is enacted within three registers, which are distinct from each other but which, through their interaction, produce meaning. Lacan calls these registers the Symbolic, the Imaginary, and the Real. Tamise Van Pelt states that the Real is not accessible to those of us who write about texts because the Real is recalcitrant to representation or symbolization, unspeakable, and resistant.[96] This is the register of sexual difference, the experience of sexed bodies that does not make sense in a way we can fully signify through language. In Lacan's famous example of the colour red through the three registers from his seminar on psychosis, he says that in the Real, red is "an aberration of perceptions."[97] The Imaginary register is the level at which the ego operates, where we make identifications with others (individuals who are identified as "small o" others) and where we construct a coherent conscious narrative of ourselves with the assistance of the ego.[98] To return to Lacan's example, in the Imaginary, red is on the plane of display, the signal of the robin's red breast to another robin to produce innate responses: as Van Pelt states, red here "is a part of a set of interrelations that provoke an understanding."[99] Finally, the Symbolic is the register of language and signification.[100] It is that which paves the way for the Imaginary, a setting for oppositional signifiers that are empty of meaning in and of themselves. Meaning is not bestowed until internalized meanings in the Imaginary and Symbolic registers are aligned: this is the Lacanian "quilting point."[101] The Symbolic is also where Lacan situates the Subject of the unconscious, which is decentred in Lacanian theory because the Subject is separate from the ego, since they inhabit the Symbolic and Imaginary registers, respectively and exclusively.[102] In the Symbolic, red is the colour of hearts and diamonds, whose only function is to oppose the black of spades and clubs in the deck of cards and as Van Pelt says, "signif[y] linguistically."[103]

Finally, the Symbolic is the register of the "big O" Other, the Other of language to whom we address our speech and who does not correspond with our "small o" others (individual people). Structurally, the Other occupies an empty place with no content, and we are aware of this. Van Pelt reminds us that in Lacan's formulation, the analyst positions themselves in the place of the big Other in order to facilitate the analysand's formulation of unconscious questions.[104] When the analyst and analysand are at the level of Symbolic interpretation, they are enacting full speech, which is in contrast to the ego's empty speech that functions to patch up imaginary inconsistencies for the purposes of achieving a unified image of the self.[105] Van Pelt states that "the logic of the image and of the imaginary register is fusional," and that "the logic of the signifier and the symbolic register is differential."[106] This means that the Imaginary register is within the level in which we make identifications and establish identities, and the Symbolic register is the level of difference within which we make binary separations. Since the Symbolic register can only express difference in binary terms, it is in this way that the Symbolic fails to capture and represent sexual difference, because sex escapes the Symbolic's significations.

Salecl argues that the contemporary subject struggles against the individualization of postmodern society. We might, then, think of the cut as a way for the subject to deal with what she defines as the deadlocks of postmodern society, which distinguish it from its pre-modern and modern manifestations. In a pre-modern society, the initiation rite establishes a sense of security with regard to one's sexual identity and provides an answer to the Symbolic structure regarding the question of gender.[107] The initiation rite also establishes the pre-modern subject as a part of a collectivity, and the law of the big Other is upheld.[108] In a modern society, Enlightenment ideals continue to uphold the status of law as the Law of the Father, and the subject seeks to establish himself or herself as a free individual by taking a stand for or against the law.[109] Once again, the Symbolic structure maintains the position of the Other. In contrast, a postmodern subject rejects and disbelieves the authority and power of the big

Other and the Symbolic structure.[110] Salecl astutely observes that this does not mean that we are completely free from a Symbolic law, but instead we are betrayed, angry, and disappointed in the fraud of the Symbolic.[111] What occurs in practices of initiation and cutting is not a response to the big Other (as it is in a pre-modern society) but rather a response to the *non-existence* of the big Other.[112] The cut is an attempt to assert the identity of the subject in relation to this absence.

Salecl identifies three Imaginary responses to the absence of the big Other in the Symbolic: narcissism, complaint, and body art. The narcissist, who is unable to form an identification with a Symbolic marker because the big Other does not exist, instead identifies with an Imaginary image or position that allows them to love themselves.[113] Another response creates what Salecl calls a "culture of complaint": one experiences an injustice or problem and thus one accuses various imaginary others of persecution and interference with one's freedom because there is no longer a belief in a symbolic order that keeps us in check.[114] While the narcissist endlessly seeks new means to perfection, to perfecting the image, the complaining subject primarily seeks financial compensation for their problems.[115] Finally, the body artist employs a perverse strategy to disavow the fact of castration[116] by ridiculing it through the spectacle. Salecl identifies these acts as ways of dealing with the postmodern condition, which is that while the Symbolic structure is still functioning, we no longer have any authorities with which we can identify. Instead we have what Salecl terms "imaginary simulacra" to identify with, or in other words, we are trapped by the endlessness of the image.[117] The body is unstable and changeable, and identity is unhinged and unfixed.

Within these conditions, the cut, as an irrevocable mark on the body, can be thought of as a way to stabilize the subject's identity on the body. The cut is the subject's protest against the demand to identify solely with "imaginary simulacra," a protest that attempts to situate the body within the ineffable Real.[118] This cut demonstrates the failure of language to represent trauma. The cut of cosmetic surgery can be thought of as a response to this trauma, a way to establish one's skin as one's own. The conditions of postmodernity described by Salecl are expressed through surfaces like the skin in a surface imagination culture. One's identity is lived through surfaces, and within cosmetic surgery narratives, the photograph occupies

the position of an ideal while the skin is de-idealized because of its inability to approximate the photograph's malleability and resiliency.

Salecl argues that skin and photographs are among the "imaginary
simulacra" we have to identify with, and these surfaces come to represent
ourselves to others. The absence of a big Other to recognize us or provide
an identificatory site leaves us floundering in the image, thus idealizing the
proliferation and choice of identities constructed around images. The
fantasy of the controllable and alterable body promised by the cosmetic
surgery industry is salient because it speaks to these imaginary simulacra
and offers a way out of the trap of one's current skin and into a new one.
A major dilemma is that these Imaginary cuts into the body are fleeting,
and only satisfy temporarily, because the image is endless and the ego is
insatiable in its desire to shore up its image-idealizations. Because of this
infinite quality of the Imaginary image, once a patient has cosmetic
surgery, she becomes surgical and is more likely to obtain other surgeries
(whether to correct the original surgery, update the original surgery, or
unrelated to the original surgery). The possibility of tailoring the skin to
one's liking is supported by the actual capacity of the photograph to
provide an image of the future skin, even though the skin is quite unlike
the photograph in its contingency.

As the interview narratives demonstrate, skin is a highly unstable
medium in cosmetic surgery. While cosmetic surgery holds out the Imaginary surface imagination fantasy of the mutable body that can be altered
at will to suit one's desires (and this is certainly a popular depiction of
cosmetic surgery), Salecl's argument about how the cut functions for the
postmodern subject as a response and protest to the absence of the
symbolic Other undermines this fantasy. While it is currently not fashionable within intellectual discourse to talk about the body as fixed, many
of the skin narratives I have explored here challenge this way of thinking.
The response to contingency by the interviewees is not to embrace it with
open arms; it is to try to mitigate its effects and control the body. The
relationship between interiority and exteriority is not challenged and
blurred, but the interviewees sought to bring them closer together in order
to assert a coherent appearance and sense of self. The marking of the
body as an object of time was not received as fluid, but rather the interviewees sought to locate their bodies within a time that they determined.
Cosmetic surgery fundamentally revolves around the cut as a protest and

response to the absence of the Other as a way to make sense of the events that happen to the body without one's will. Becoming concerned with the "imaginary simulacra" of life is fundamentally about positioning the image as an identificatory site, a situation that the cosmetic surgery industry capitalizes on.

The interview narratives document the impossibility of stopping up psychic distress through Imaginary means that support the ego's identifications and narratives. Psychic distress is no longer conceptualized at the level of interiority, but is exteriorized onto the skin's surface (or photographic surface) where it can be moulded and shaped by cosmetic surgeons. These Imaginary interventions temporarily and partially address the symptom of being in a body that one does not want to be in, but because the intervention is at the Imaginary level, the symptom will reappear in another location. Through surface imagining that the distress is caused at the level of the skin, and rendering the skin closer to the photograph through the cut-protest, the cosmetic surgery patient finds a partial satisfaction that coincides with the ideals and norms of her culture. The proliferation of cosmetic surgery in contemporary Western cultures specifically, and the power of surface imaginations more broadly, can be understood as an effect of the demand to exist on the Imaginary plane through self-fashioning and image creation, as an Imaginary manifestation of control over one's body. This infinite capacity for change aligns well with the neoliberal valorization of choice in Western advanced capitalist societies of the late twentieth and early twenty-first century, which promote the individualization of suffering that originates in the social and cultural. As I explore in the conclusion to this book, the narratives described here express a tension between these fantasies of transformation and the wish for somatic stability and comfort. This is a tension that starkly reveals the limits of surface imagination, as well as the limits to the promises made by the cosmetic surgery industry.

CONCLUSION

5

A culture that counts cosmetic surgeries within its scope of
legitimate medical procedures is a culture in which the
landscapes[1] of *all* of our bodies are fundamentally altered.
In this milieu, bodies come to be seen as mutable and plastic raw material, to be shaped by our own fantasies, desires, and imaginations. The cosmetic surgery industry markets itself as limitless in its
scope and talent, relying on photographic representations to do the work
of convincing the viewer that her own skin will mirror the photograph's
surface. This is surface imagination in operation: the dual surfaces studied in this book – the photographic and the dermal – are collapsed into
each other to fantasize dramatic personal change through transforming
the body's surface. Whether or not one has the means to access cosmetic
surgeries, the pervasiveness of representations and narratives of cosmetic
surgery means that we can still imagine transforming our own bodies, as
well as the bodies of others. These exterior interventions are conceptualized as interventions into identity, a narrative that is enabled by the primacy of surface imaginations. The body that is open to transformation
imagines identity as subject to modification according to current social,
economic, and political trends. The transformation of identity is also
expected to align with projects that make the self more marketable and
appealing to others in the public sphere. The intractability of the body is
disavowed and becomes a source of frustration and personal failure. To

conclude this deliberation on cosmetic surgery, photography, and skin, I want to think through the implications of surface imagination for contemporary conceptualizations of embodiment.

My concept of surface imagination is connected to Eva Illouz's concept of emotional capitalism, which also troubles the boundaries between interior/exterior and private/public. Emotional capitalism challenges the assumption that capitalism is fully rational and a-emotional, and instead maintains that "an intensely specialized emotional culture" emerged concurrently with capitalism.[2] Illouz argues that emotional styles and techniques of relating to others generated within capitalist discourses came to be employed both in the middle-class nuclear family and in the workplace. These emotional styles and techniques were similar and strongly emphasized the conscious management and discipline of emotions.[3] Thus, the private self was self-fashioned through public performance and tethered to understandings of everyday life generated from the public sphere, particularly the realms of economics and politics. This intimate affiliation between the public and the private spheres, bonded together through common emotional techniques and styles, relies on the conceptualization of the self as a project to be worked on in the workplace and the home. Learning techniques of controlling and demonstrating appropriate emotional expression, sometimes in conflict with one's actual emotional expression – particularly when that expression is conceived of as "negative," in the cases of anger, frustration, and sadness – is conceived as a marketable skill inside the workplace and the home. Emotional capitalism thus coincides with surface imagination, because in a culture shaped by surface imagination and emotional capitalism, the emphasis is on the self-presentation of emotions to others as an ongoing life project. Contemporary cosmetic surgery, structured by surface imagination fantasies that revolve around the self as capital in the public and the private spheres, can be understood as a corporeal way of managing emotions within an emotional capitalist culture that produces subjects conceived of as marketable products. Within the culture of cosmetic surgery, emotions are negotiated and managed on the surface of the body and through surface representations like photographs.

In its early stages, this book emerged from a persistent concern that feminist research about beauty and femininity consistently failed to speak to the myriad investments women held in feminine beauty practices, including cosmetic surgery. To conflate the ideologies of the beauty and cosmetic surgery industries with the motivations of individual women to participate in beauty and cosmetic surgery practices is to make a dangerous and flawed assumption. This type of analysis leads to narrow and unsubtle understandings of the meaning of cosmetic surgery in women's lives. The assumption that women who undergo cosmetic surgery are wholly, unproblematically, and uncritically in support of the cosmetic surgery industry trivializes their experiences, as well as an interest in beauty. It is easy to dismiss beauty as politically insignificant, and to portray women who have cosmetic surgery as ridiculous and vain; many will embrace such a critique enthusiastically because of overt or internalized misogyny, whether they identify as feminist or not. Further, this critique misses the opportunity to consider what it might mean for contemporary understandings of embodiment that, in cosmetic surgery cultures structured by surface imagination, emotions are negotiated through the skin and the photograph, rather than through the subject's interior.

I have been presenting my research on cosmetic surgery at academic conferences since May 2005. Time and again, I am approached by my feminist colleagues with comments that express disgust and disbelief over the existence of cosmetic surgery procedures: for example, "I just don't understand how someone could do something like *that* to their body!" This response fascinates me in its blurring together of repulsion and empathy, and its deep-rooted gut origins in an imagining of the painful embodied experiences of the cutting, penetration, and burning of skin, flesh, and bone for an aesthetic result. This response establishes difference and distance between the cosmetic surgery patient and the speaker[4] through rendering the cosmetic surgery patient pathological due to her willingness to bear corporeal suffering for physical beauty. This response, finally, is entrenched in a critique of cosmetic surgery that is wholly social and cannot comprehend what surgery might do for an individual who suffers from her bodily morphology.[5] This social critique suggests that if we can adequately gain mastery over our minds, we will no longer require surgery because we will be sufficiently enlightened and able to change others to think as "we" do. While I recognize that this is a bit of a caricature of social critiques of femininity, beauty, and cosmetic surgery, at its broadest level of inquiry this book project seeks to challenge this critique using individual narratives of cosmetic surgery and psychoanalytic theory to theorize attachments to beauty and femininity from a feminist perspective.

I agree with Alessandra Lemma that we are deceiving ourselves if we assume that a distance exists between the horrified speaker and the cosmetic surgery patient. Lemma suggests that Botox injections and anti-wrinkle creams exist on a continuum, rather than in separate fields.[6] What links together these various practices is the seductive quality of these possible responses, a seductive quality connected to the ongoing project of daily body modification (wearing makeup, for example) and episodic body modification (undergoing cosmetic surgery, for example). The development of surface imagination as a concept is a method of showing the connections between the practices that exist along Lemma's proposed continuum, as well as a response to these types of horrified reactions from feminists. Surface imagination explains the fantasy of self-transformation – a body that can be controlled and manipulated according to one's desire, with a result that will sink into the skin and lead to long-lasting psychical change as well. This is a highly seductive fantasy in a culture of emotional capitalism. Being able to comprehend and distinguish surface imagination fantasies and seductions can, as Lemma says, contribute to "know[ing] something about our own experience of being-in-a-body and of being, inevitably, the object of the other's gaze."[7] I would go further, however, to say that these recognitions and understandings are not just individual projects, but a project of understanding and recognizing our society and culture.

As I argued in the introduction to this book, surface imagination is a concept well suited to analyse cosmetic surgery and other body modification practices, yet it goes beyond these because the idea that we create identity through transforming surfaces in our lives can be applied to many different cultural phenomena. My hope is that theorizing surface imaginations can allow researchers and other observers and critics of contemporary cultures to remain deeply critical of cosmetic surgery as an industry yet sympathetic with and connected to the patients' experiences of cosmetic surgery. I maintain that ethically, we must take cosmetic surgery patients seriously when they claim that transforming their body's surface has had a profound impact on their identities and lives.

Admittedly, attempting to maintain a critique of the cosmetic surgery industry alongside empathy for individuals who undergo cosmetic surgery is an ambitious and sometimes contradictory project. The cosmetic surgery industry is informed by an ideology and history that is deeply disturbing in its attachments to racist and sexist ideals of feminine beauty;

on the other hand, the industry comprises various individuals who may or may not hold perspectives consistent with these discourses. Likewise, in the field of cosmetic surgery studies, there are countless examples of individual patients navigating the industry in ways that challenge dominant narratives; however, this is not to deny that there are individual patients who desire to conform to mainstream beauty ideals structured by racism and sexism. As a theorist studying an industry and experience that is itself full of contradictions, I must maintain these paradoxes. As discussed in chapter 1, several scholars within the field of feminist cosmetic surgery studies have sided too much with one pole (critique/misogyny) or the other (empathy/agency).

Further, we must resist the Cartesian impulse to subordinate body to mind, or in the terms of this book, surface to depth. Focusing my argument on the surface is not to say that contemporary Western conceptualizations of embodiment are "superficial," that is, trivial; it is to say instead that surface is the primary site upon which identity is negotiated and transformed and thus surface matters very deeply. This emphasis is also a way of exposing the limits and lacunae of surface imagination, because the fantasies and seductions of surface imagination cultures attempt to place the subject on a two-dimensional plane in order to present the subject as whole and invulnerable. This erasure of everyday vulnerability and fragmentation in favour of episodic indomitability and wholeness needs to be revealed, because in a surface imagination culture vulnerability and fragmentation are explained as failures of the individual rather than as failures of the fantasy or seduction.

My decision to incorporate psychoanalytic theory into this inquiry into cosmetic surgery and to craft a psychoanalytic methodological lens for interview narrative analysis is founded on a conviction that psychoanalysis is precisely what we need to think through interrogative statements like, "I just don't understand how someone could *do* something like *that* to their body!" This layer of analysis allows us to reflect on both the manifest and latent content in cosmetic surgery narratives; the question of why one might have surgery for aesthetic reasons even though it seems illogical to some; and finally, the question of what psychical structures, fantasies, and seductions operate within the patient's experience, as well as her relationships to her self, her surgeon, and her others. Cosmetic surgery *is* troubling; for some this is because many procedures require patients to accept death as a rare though entirely possible outcome, and for others it is because the industry exploits insecurities and oppressions rooted in social relations of gender and race in particular for profit. As I have explored in this book, the patient who seeks out cosmetic surgery finds herself confronted with forced choices and coerced relationships within the profession. If we consider the fact that many patients are required to sign waivers that indicate they are aware that they could die during or as a result of their surgery, we are faced with a very serious consequence of cosmetic surgery – the death of the patient. This alone ought to be reason enough to take patient stories and motivations seriously, rather than dismissing them as superficial or motivated by vanity. Attempting to achieve surface imagination fantasies through cosmetic surgery is not a puerile or shallow pursuit; it can be, for some, a life and death question.

While conducting my research, I felt great empathy with the women I interviewed, as well as the millions of others who engage with the North American cosmetic surgery industry each year in order to change a part or parts of their bodies.[8] The challenges and successes of this engagement are varied; while some will find satisfaction and attain a desired result, some will encounter profound dissatisfaction through engaging with an industry that inherently promotes gendered, racist, and fatphobic ideals of human bodies, and some will find a blended satisfaction and dissatisfaction (as many of my interviewees reported). For this reason, I cannot agree with Kathy Davis that cosmetic surgery enables the patient to become an "embodied subject" through her "agency" within the process. The process of cosmetic surgery is profoundly objectifying, and this objectification emanates not just from the cultural context, but also from the surgeon and the patient herself because all three of these dimensions and agents in the experience, industry, and practice of cosmetic surgery are structured by surface imagination fantasies. While the patient does have agency insofar as she elects to have cosmetic surgery and is thus not coerced into the procedure, the patient does not have the agency to dictate under which conditions she will have surgery, and the gatekeeping surgeon does not permit full and unmediated access to surgery. Consider the difficulties ORLAN faced in seeking a cosmetic surgeon to assist her in achieving her surgical vision, noted in the preface to this book. One of the major obstacles to achieving her artistic vision was establishing and retaining control as the patient, author, and artist of her surgeries, while the surgeon occupied the place of medium or tool. The gatekeeping performed by the cosmetic surgery industry limits the scope and breadth of surgical possibilities available to the patient, which is in stark contrast to the infinite fantasies of surface imagination offered by the cosmetic surgery industry. Patients must thus negotiate between surface imagination expectations, produced by photographs, that cosmetic surgery can completely revamp the body to look like whatever ideal one might desire, and the limits imposed by the contingent and unpredictable skin, as well as by the gatekeepers of the cosmetic surgery industry. The skin is the embodied boundary that marks the limits of cosmetic surgery possibilities, while the photograph is deployed to promise boundless and disembodied transformation.

Fortunately, many patients are able to get what they want from this objectifying process, and indeed all the women I interviewed indicated that they were happy with the outcomes of their surgeries. Most offered solid evidence of the ways that their lives had improved after their surgeries, such as career advancement (Nicanor), sexual empowerment (Tonya and Melinda), feeling youthful and alive (Tigerlily), and being comfortable in their own skins (Leah and Victoria). However, most also commented on how the process of attaining these results was less than perfect; for example, months-long numbness (Tigerlily), dismissive surgeons (Tonya and Leah), severe reactions to anaesthesia and pain medication that required additional hospitalization (Melinda), being unconvinced that the treatment was working (Victoria), and being unsatisfied with results just three months post-surgery (Diana). Analysing the interview narratives using poetic transcription and psychoanalytic theory allowed me to construct a critique of the cosmetic surgery profession that holds on to the tensions between the benefits received by those who have cosmetic surgery and the dystopic sexist and racist conditions under which the profession operates. This tensive relationship can further be understood as the unlimited promises of the photograph coming into conflict with the limits of the skin; this is precisely the conflict between cosmetic surgery as an industry founded on the seductiveness of surface imagination fantasies and cosmetic surgery as a practice that can have various outcomes – positive, negative, and ambivalent – for individual patients.

Further, psychoanalytic theory offers a theoretical framework to develop new methodologies that can better represent the effects and structures of surface imaginations. Poetic transcription borrows from surface imagination in its emphasis on the formal, stylistic manipulations of language, and yet, unlike many cultural products of surface imaginations, does not do violence through erasure of one or more parts, denial of the fixed or stable, insistence on wholeness, or demand for endless reinvention and documentation of the transformation. Poetic transcription can hold open the tension between surface imagination violence (the cosmetic surgery industry, in this book) and surface imagination outcomes (patient experiences and the practice of cosmetic surgery). Without the support of metaphors like the bodily ego and skin ego, and the concept of the unconscious, these kinds of methodological innovations are unintelligible. These metaphors and concepts expose an aperture in surface imagination narratives of cosmetic surgery, and they provide models for an embodied language or presentation of language that does not attempt to close this gap but instead keeps it open. This is the opposite action of the cosmetic surgery industry's surface imagination fantasies and stories, which seek to seduce by attempting to close the aperture through erasing the impossibility of fully realizing these fantasies.

Cosmetic surgery mobilizes the fantasy of the mutable body, which includes the desire to alleviate psychic suffering through the body itself, as well as the desire for a body that is impermeable and controllable. This fantasy is called a *surface imagination fantasy* because it is structured by surface imagination: the belief and hope that a change to the exterior can enhance or improve the interior, and further, that the outside creates and is more significant than the inside. The fantasized body in surface imagination cultures is a body that can be contained, and the surface imagination seduction of cosmetic surgery is that the body is infinitely transformable and thus controllable. The body that is open to transformation is premised on a particularly North American conceptualization of identity that imagines identity as subject to modification according to current social, economic, and political trends. Tethering the idea that changing the body can change our emotional and personal lives to the notion that we need to be able to remake ourselves in order to be competitive and desirable in love, work, and life creates a cultural milieu in which cosmetic surgery can flourish. And as this book shows, the cosmetic surgery industry has been adept at manipulating its cultural conditions from the beginning through emphasizing psychological over beauty outcomes.

Photography sustains this surface imagination fantasy of the mutable body, and supports the practice of cosmetic surgery through fragmentation and transformation of the body image. Looking at a body through the perspective of the cosmetic surgeon is much like looking at a body through the lens of the camera; and likewise, the photographic editor looks at the body in the same way a surgeon might. Photographs offer inspiration to cosmetic surgery patients by providing many examples of bodily configurations that are desirable in a contemporary context, or by providing evidence of the more desirable past of one's body. Whether an alteration happens through the skin, flesh, and bone or through photo retouching, the effect on the image printed on photographic paper appears virtually the same. Because we live in a photographically and visually oriented culture, the difference between photo and surgical retouching is negligible. Indeed, I am fully convinced by Virginia Blum's argument that cosmetic surgery prepares the body to be photographed. Many, if not most cosmetic surgeries make the body and face look good in clothing and accessories, though underneath the clothes and beyond the hairline, the damage to the body is often very apparent. Cosmetic surgery alleviates some degree of psychic suffering, and it does so through the visual realm of the surface. What can be seen becomes more significant than what can be felt. So, while the de-idealized skin surface of cosmetic surgery bears the marks and other side effects of surgery that must be concealed and negotiated, this is not as important as the favourable results upon the idealized photographic surface.

This visual realm is the realm of surface. Skin is the material and metaphorical site upon which the fantasies of cosmetic surgery and photography are enacted. As a location where the cultural and social meet interior life, the skin is also the landscape upon which this surface imagination drama unfolds. Cosmetic surgery hopes to emulate the miraculous attributes of skin, not just to reverse time (as Steven Connor argues) but also to offer a container and permeable barrier to hold psychical contents and re-establish or experiment with psychical boundaries. The skin in cosmetic surgery exists in anterior time as well, and patients and surgeons are seduced by the photograph's possibilities that help project the skin into its future existence. Gender and race in particular are projected onto and read off of the skin. In terms of skin and femininity, sometimes this marking can threaten one's feminine self (in the case of wrinkles, acne, and loss of breast tissue post-pregnancy/lactation), or it can serve as an unwanted marking of femininity upon the skin (in the case of stretch marks). An intervention into the skin through cosmetic surgery is a way of asserting a desired control over the body with the hope of alleviating suffering through the skin.

So, what is it that cosmetic surgery accomplishes psychically and socially in a surface imagination culture? While happiness has ostensibly remained the dominant psychical outcome of cosmetic surgery since the mid-1800s, this word does not capture what is at stake in cosmetic surgery, either individually or culturally. In the final analysis, I am left with the tensions between postmodern fantasies of a mutable body that is capable of infinite change and the narratives of the interviewees, which express hope that cosmetic surgery would effect a permanent change that would fix the body.[9] Silverman notes that while we may possess a certain openness to a nomadic narrative life, we are recalcitrant to changes in our bodily morphology, particularly when these changes are not culturally esteemed.[10] Thus we either seek to maintain our body in its present state, or we want to make it better than it is by conforming more closely to a culturally venerated image. While it is the case that those who undergo cosmetic surgery will likely have more surgery, this has less to do with an endlessly transformable body than it does with a desire to secure the body within a particular configuration that is usually rooted in a chronologically past or fantasmatic body.

In her reading of Cindy Sherman's *Untitled Film Stills,* Silverman invokes the psychoanalytic concept of the "good enough." This concept emerges from Donald Winnicott's work as he describes the "good enough" mother who offers a measured response to the infant's needs. If the mother were to respond to all of the infant's needs, the infant would be suffocated, and if the mother were to respond to few of the infant's needs, the infant would be neglected. Thus, the "good enough" mother dynamically adapts to the infant's demands, and her responses lessen as the infant is able to endure frustration and the mother's inability to respond to every need.[11] Silverman uses this concept to think through our identificatory positions in relation to Sherman's photographs, and she suggests that we identify with the women themselves rather than with their ideal imagos.[12] We see the women in Sherman's photographs posing in a manner that aspires to measure up to a culturally revered image of femininity. Because the makeup, costuming, lighting, staging, and exterior props are so central and obvious to the photographs, Silverman argues that the women in Sherman's *Untitled Film Stills* are able to effect a "good enough" approximation of their ideal imagos.[13] Silverman's citation of the "good enough" approximation of femininity suggests that the women in Sherman's photographs take on femininity in a way that is provisional and does not attempt to fill the space from which desire springs. The possible identifications that these photographs might inspire are shaped by the experiences of being embodied and being seen by others.

In the introduction to her study of body modification, Lemma identifies two concerns that we all face: first, that we are all in a body; and second, that we are subject to the gaze of the other.[14] Her study of body modification is concerned with why some individuals deal with psychic conflicts through the body, rather than through narrative. Further, she wants to understand what makes some use the body to address psychic conflicts in a pathological manner. These concerns are similar to Silverman's in her examination of Sherman's work; more importantly, the attempt to resolve psychic conflicts through the skin is produced by surface imagination fantasies structured by the seductive possibilities of transformation. Through her diverse work in private psychoanalytic practice, public mental health service provision in prisons and other institutions, and as a consultant to reality television makeover shows in the UK, Lemma identifies three dominant unconscious fantasies of body modification practices. The first is the "reclaiming phantasy," the taking back of the self from a foreign presence that lives in the body (she also calls this an "expulsion phantasy"); the second is the "perfect match phantasy," which is the approximation of an ideal body that will secure love and desire from the other; and the third is the "self-made phantasy," which is an attack on the object envious of the subject's independence through proving that the self can make itself and is free from dependence.[15] There is a privileging of depth implicit in her analysis because, while she acknowledges that the surface of our bodies will narrate that which we cannot speak, she also claims that there is something "under the skin" that is more profound, presumably the internal world of psychic life. Her analysis of body modifications like cosmetic surgery is thus very different from mine, which privileges surface; however, the trajectories of our work are complementary and support each other. Lemma argues that coming to an understanding of the unconscious phantasy behind body modification practices can help those patients who find body modification compelling and necessary. I argue that understanding surface imagination fantasies can aid our understanding of identity as fashioned through surfaces, an analysis that weaves together the cultural with the individual. The intersections and contradictions between these different understandings of surface body modifications emerge from our singular locations of praxis: one individual, one cultural.

Initially, I imagined an extension of the "good enough" approximation of idealized femininity that could apply to the function of cosmetic surgery; however, I take Silverman's caution that the concept of "good enough" might be easily incorporated into an agenda that promotes an unbridled agency that misunderstands the good enough as acceptance of failure.[16] Perhaps a utopic vision of cosmetic surgery could put forth the practice as a means to approximate a "good enough" configuration of one's body. On the other hand, my research has demonstrated that while cosmetic surgery carries many psychic benefits, perhaps most importantly the alignment of the visual imago and the proprioceptive ego, any engagement with the profession is far from utopic. While the motivations expressed by the interviewees are easily understandable, since most of the interviewees became comfortable in their own skins and in their relationships with others, the interviewees were confronted with imperfect options resulting from the photographically dominated mandate of the cosmetic surgery profession. Their narratives push up against the limits of the seductive promises of surface imagination understandings of cosmetic surgery, which attempt to present the body as whole and impenetrable. The interviewees negotiated both a profession that slates all participants into rigidly gendered roles with few options for surgical outcomes and a cultural context that trivializes femininity and beauty. And as a consequence, even though the interviewees were overall satisfied with the results of their surgeries, the complaints present in their narratives denoted by scars, numbness, and flaws in their outcomes are indeed registered as necessary failures that are nonetheless a worthwhile compromise for attaining a surgical objective. This is the compromise of surface imagination, where the result is incomplete and not totally fulfilling in contrast to the fantasized body promised by the cosmetic surgery industry, and yet it is also because of surface imagination that the imperfect results are indeed so satisfying.

APPENDIX: INTERVIEWEES

NAME	AGE	ETHNICITY*	SURGERY AND AGE AT TIME OF SURGERY
Tigerlily	75	German	Face, neck, and eye lift, 67
Melinda	30	Caucasian	Breast augmentation, 27
Leah	25	(none given)	Breast reduction, 24
Tonya	29	White	Breast reduction, 21
Diana	35	White	Liposuction, 35
Nicanor	67	Hispano-American	Face and eye lift, 46
Victoria	25	Jewish	Chemical peels and laser treatments of face for acne, ongoing from age 24

*The interviewees chose the terms for their ethnicity.

A NOTE ON THE COVER

The Photograph

The photograph on the cover, *Beauty Recovery Room 002, 23 years old, Seoul, South Korea*, 2013, is one of a series of photographs by Ji Yeo of young women recovering from cosmetic surgery. The cosmetic surgery industry in South Korea is robust and expanding; indeed, according to the Society of Aesthetic Plastic Surgery in 2010, it has the highest per capita rate of elective cosmetic procedures in the world, and cosmetic surgery is normalized as a routine component of body maintenance and improvement.[1] In her artist's statement for the work, Yeo highlights that each of the women has already undergone surgeries and has plans for future surgeries, due to the cultural value of being beautiful in Korea. *Beauty Recovery Room* has been featured in several popular media outlets, and the series is on Yeo's website: http://jiyeo.com/the-beauty/.

The women that I interviewed and that Yeo photographed live in different national contexts, yet they all grapple with surface imagination fantasies of embodiment. When I first came across Ji Yeo's *Beauty Recovery Room*, the parallels between her work and mine struck me. The subjects of these photographs are arresting; they invite the viewer in to the uncomfortable feeling of living in a body, a personal discomfort amplified by structural relations of oppression. The reader will notice several of this book's themes, narratives, and counter-narratives in its cover photograph. Yeo uses photography, the medium used to fashion idealized skins, to disrupt the surface imagination fantasies of the cosmetic surgery industry. The photograph is disquieting because it is a rupture in the seamlessness of cosmetic surgery's before and after fantasy, exposing an in-between moment of banality, discomfort, and boredom. Hugged tightly by bandages, the woman in this image reminds me of Diana's second skin composed of women's foundation garments, as well as Tigerlily's futile search for images of healing. She is captivating to me because she resists the demand to face the camera and smile after cosmetic surgery. Instead, this woman's image consummately embodies the compromise of cosmetic surgery as a way of living more comfortably in one's body that is determined by the parameters of an industry that can be very limiting. I am deeply grateful for her resilience and vulnerability, and for Ji Yeo's permission to reproduce the photograph.

The Artist

Ji Yeo is a New York-based artist who pursued her master's degree in photography at Rhode Island School of Design as a president's scholarship and Henry Wolf Scholarship awardee. She graduated from Seoul National University in Seoul, South Korea in visual communication design and studied at the International Center of Photography in New York, USA. Her work is held in collections at The Smithsonian and Rhode Island School of Design Museum and has been shown at the International Center of Photography in New York, National Portrait Gallery in London, ClampArt in New York, Houston Center for Photography in Houston, and Scottish National Portrait Gallery in Glasgow. Her work has been featured worldwide by the BBC UK, *Guardian* UK, BBC Brazil, *Huffington Post, National Geographic Proof,* LA *Times reFramed, Daily Mail* UK, *Wired Magazine, Dazed Digital, Marie Claire* Brazil, *Esquire* Russia, *Blink magazine, Von magazine International,* and many others.

PREFACE

1 ORLAN, personal website.
2 ORLAN, quoted in Jill O'Bryan, *Carnal Art*, 19.
3 Virginia Blum, *Flesh Wounds*.
4 ORLAN, "The Future of the Body."
5 Ibid.
6 Ibid.
7 Ibid.
8 Ibid.
9 Ibid.
10 While "The Reincarnation of Saint ORLAN" initially proposed a surgery to construct a huge "phallophanic" nose as its endpoint, cosmetic surgeons refused to perform this surgery and ORLAN's medical adviser discouraged it because it would have altered ORLAN's voice and posed too many physical risks and complications. Thus, ORLAN's body never reached the endpoint, the goal each cosmetic surgery patient desires, and instead exists in the ambiguous in-between space that is both rejected and used for fantasmatic projection in cosmetic surgery. I discuss this status of "forever becoming" a body in ORLAN's work in chapter 3.
11 Rachel Armstrong, "Anger, Art and Medicine," 173.
12 Ibid.
13 All names given are pseudonyms chosen by the interviewees. Further, all identifying information has been changed in order to protect the anonymity of the interviewees.
14 There are many examples of these claims, particularly in the "testimonials" sections of doctor's websites. For example, the website of Toronto surgeon Dr Martin Jugenburg features patient testimonies with comments such as, "I literally feel like a new woman," "The work you have done on me has truly changed my life," "His work has allowed me to be much more confident and more outgoing," and "Like I've always said love who you are and if there's something you want to improve upon go for it. This is your life. Your story. Your day. Never mind what others may say or not say. Make at least one chapter of your life a memorable one." Jugenberg, "Dr Martin Jugenberg Reviews."
15 Hurst, "Surgical Stories, Gendered Telling."

MAKING INTRODUCTIONS

1 The fastest growing procedures in the cosmetic surgery market are those that are relatively inexpensive, non-invasive, and can be performed by non-medical doctors, such as skin treatments like Victoria's, but also injectables like Botox (to paralyze small muscles to reduce the appearance of wrinkles) and Restylane (a "filler" used for lip enhancement and wrinkle reduction). Later I discuss how Victoria's interview fits and doesn't fit within the interviews as a whole.

CHAPTER ONE

1 The following are some recent studies on the psychological benefits of cosmetic surgery for patients that indicate positive psychological outcomes post-surgery. Interestingly, Von Soest et al. (2011) note that a limitation of most studies is that they generally occur within twelve months after a surgery: Von Soest et al., "Psychosocial Changes after Cosmetic Surgery"; Von Soest et al., "The Effects of Cosmetic Surgery"; Sarwer et al., "Two-Year Results"; Kosowski et al., "A Systematic Review"; and Dowling et al., "Psychological Characteristics and Outcomes."

2 Feminist scholarship on cosmetic surgery has gained such currency in contemporary understandings of the practice that Fraser analysed feminist scholarship alongside women's magazines, medical literature, and regulatory material in order to understand common meanings about gender and cosmetic surgery that circulate among these major discourses (see Fraser, *Cosmetic Surgery, Gender and Culture*). The summaries found in Gimlin, *Cosmetic Surgery Narratives,* 56–68 and Jones, *Skintight,* 18–29 are particularly good, thorough, and recent. Heyes and Jones have edited an excellent collection of texts representative of the past and present of the field in their *Cosmetic Surgery: A Feminist Primer.*

3 Davis, *Reshaping the Female Body,* 5.

4 Bordo, "Material Girl," 337.

5 For more on fashion and cosmetic surgery, particularly how the skin has been conceived of as a textile in cosmetic surgery, see Hurst, "The Skin-Textile in Cosmetic Surgery."

6 Holliday and Sanchez Taylor claim that feminist analyses of cosmetic surgery set up a binary between the surgically modified (artificial) body and the non-modified (natural) body, reproducing narratives of false beauty that are well known through masculinist philosophies of feminine beauty and popular culture (Holliday and Sanchez Taylor, "Aesthetic Surgery as False Beauty," 189). The result is that the non-surgically modified body is championed as a form of resistance. Several earlier feminist works on cosmetic surgery reproduce these

approaches. For example, Morgan describes cosmetic surgery as a technological invasion of women's bodies that is becoming normalized in "Women and the Knife," and argues for a feminist utopian version of cosmetic surgery that valorizes ugliness and inscribes wrinkles into the skin and injects fat into the body. Balsamo argues that despite the promises of cosmetic surgery, the practice reifies conventional gender norms through a normalizing technological gaze in "On the Cutting Edge." In "The Confession Mirror" Spitzack writes of cosmetic surgery as a form of technological cultural control over women's bodies, defining the female body as flawed and in need of surgical "fixing," which involves discipline and surveillance of the female body. Sobchack's "Scary Women" examines the relationship between cinematic images of women's bodies and cosmetic surgery, and she also champions a resistant approach to beauty and cosmetic surgery by valuing and accepting her aging face and body. In addition, there are more contemporary works that draw on these approaches. For example, Jeffreys' 2005 *Beauty and Misogyny* argues that the UN definition of a harmful traditional/cultural practice is biased in favour of the West, so that practices like makeup and cosmetic surgery are not listed as harmful practices even though they fit within the UN definition (3), and that cosmetic surgery is "self-mutilation by proxy" (150).

7 Gimlin's analysis in *Body Work* adopts a similar approach. She argues that women who undergo cosmetic surgery do so as a way of "making do" in a culture that is highly judgmental of women based on appearance. In contrast to Davis, however, Gimlin is more critical of the narratives offered to her by interviewees, stating that "women who undergo plastic surgery help to reproduce some of the worst aspects of the beauty culture, not so much through the act of the surgery itself as through their ideological efforts to restore appearance as an indicator of character" (108).

8 Davis, *Reshaping the Female Body*, 175–7.

9 For an example of this critique, see Gimlin, *Cosmetic Surgery Narratives*, 63.

10 Davis, *Reshaping the Female Body*, 5.

11 Huss-Ashmore, "'The Real Me,'" 36.

12 Blum, *Flesh Wounds*, 49.

13 Heyes, *Self-Transformations*, 22.

14 Jones, *Skintight*, 12.

15 Gimlin, *Cosmetic Surgery Narratives*, 101–2.

16 Ibid., 101.

17 Ibid., 101–2.

18 Edmond's *Pretty Modern*, an ethnography of *plástica* (cosmetic surgery) in Brazil, provides an insightful analysis of the practice that offers much material for future cross-cultural comparative analyses.

19 Wegenstein, *The Cosmetic Gaze*, 2.

20 Ibid., ix.

21 Ibid., 109.

22 Ibid., 186. The concept of the "cosmetic gaze" has the advantage of being more nuanced than Laura Mulvey's "male gaze," (Mulvey, "Visual Pleasure and Narrative Cinema") and permits an understanding of cinema and art that can reveal the various "machinic sutures" that operate in these realms (152).

23 See Cheng, *Second Skin*; Gilman, *Creating Beauty to Cure the Soul*; Gilman, *Making the Body Beautiful*; and Haiken, *Venus Envy*.

24 Jones, *Skintight*, 159.

25 Scholars informed by interdisciplinary cultural studies have attempted to take up this gap in their work. Jones claims that "makeover culture" reveals the space that exists in between the before and after photographs that are ubiquitous in cosmetic surgery culture. She argues that through representing the during of cosmetic surgery, the violence of cosmetic surgery "become[s] acceptable via the screen" (*Skintight*, 52). I would qualify this claim by emphasizing that the in-between space that is revealed is heavily edited, sanitized, and made more palatable. Jones herself notes this, although she concludes that even though these in-between images are highly mediated in *Extreme Makeover*, they are accurate enough to facilitate an interest in and engagement with the during spaces of cosmetic surgery (Ibid., 159). I am not, however, fully convinced that these sequences have a significant influence on the seduction of the before and after structures of transformation in cosmetic surgery.

26 Isaacs' "The Nature and Function of Fantasy" outlines this distinction very clearly.

27 Žižek, *Looking Awry*, 6.

28 For example, Davis comments that when she observed fifty-five consultation appointments with patients seeking cosmetic surgery, she was able to tell what kind of surgery the patient was seeking in only one instance; further, her suspicions of what surgery a patient was seeking were frequently proven wrong. Davis, *Reshaping the Female Body*, 70.

29 Most interview-based research demonstrates this claim. For one of the first interview-based studies that demonstrates this, see Davis, *Reshaping the Female Body*.

30 The following are excellent explications of this: Lloyd, *The Man of Reason* and Spelman, "Woman as Body."

31 See Frueh, *Swooning Beauty*.

32 Cheng, *Second Skins*, 167–8. This devaluation and ignorance of the relationship between being and surface is especially detrimental, according to Cheng, since "when it comes to representations of women and racial minorities, the visual is almost always negatively inflected

and usually seen as a tool of commoditization and objectification"
(168). Cheng argues that in the early twentieth century there is a "ten-
sile and delicate moment," seen in the relationship between modernist
style and entertainer Josephine Baker, that reveals "profound engagements with and reimagings of the relationship between interiority and
exteriority, between essence and covering" (11). Thus, surface and
essence are signifiers that co-constitute each other; according to
Cheng, Josephine Baker's black skin is a surface that exposes a "crisis
of visuality" as she is inchoately both fetishized (and fully knowable)
and existent as a subversive subject who "disappear[s] into appearance" (171–2).

33 In chapter 4, I explore this shift historically through the work of
    Benthien.

34 Meiners, "Inquiries into the Regulation of Disordered Bodies," 3.

35 But perhaps a liar-bird?

36 Trinh, *Framer/Framed*, 95.

37 Ibid., 73.

38 Narayan and George, "Personal and Folk Narrative," 454.

39 Trinh, *Framer/Framed*, 138.

40 Ibid., 138.

41 Bourdieu, *In Other Words*, 60.

42 I do not use these concepts in my analysis of cosmetic surgery, and
    will not define them here. The ego and abjection are concepts belong-
    ing to the conscious realm, while the death drive and repetition com-
    pulsion exist within the field of the unconscious. For full definitions,
    see Callard, "The Taming of Psychoanalysis."

43 Ibid., 308.

44 Ibid., 298.

45 Kvale, "The Psychoanalytic Interview," 89.

46 Thomas, "The Implications of Psychoanalysis," 543.

47 In fact, I myself have done this in the past!

48 Roseneil, "The Ambivalences of Angel's 'Arrangement,'" 865. In
    claiming that all sociological analyses are interpretive, Roseneil gives
    the example of common categories of demographic analysis (for ex-
    ample, "working class," "person of colour") used repeatedly in soci-
    ology that often do not correspond to research subjects' own
    self-identifications. At first glance this seems to be a rather flimsy ex-
    ample; however, I think it is more profound than that and demon-
    strates how the way we "organize" people in research can alienate
    these subjects. If I categorize a group of people as "working class," a
    label recognizable to other academics but not those within that group,
    how meaningful is it as a category of analysis?

49 Ibid., 866.

50 Hunt, *Psychoanalytic Aspects of Fieldwork*, 13. This is not to say that

other methodologies do not also consider the self in this manner (ethnography being one of the major examples).

51 Ibid., 27.
52 Ibid., 29.
53 Ibid., 62.
54 This is what Freud would call "wild analysis."
55 For more on grounded theory approaches, see Glaser and Strauss, *The Discovery of Grounded Theory*; Clarke, *Situational Analysis*; and Charmaz, *Constructing Grounded Theory*.
56 Shostak, *Interviewing and Representation*, 3–4.
57 Many thanks are owed to Kristine Klement and Shawn Thompson, who articulated this definition so clearly as I struggled to explain it.
58 Lacan, quoted in Lather, *Getting Smart*, 9.
59 Callard, "The Taming of Psychoanalysis," 307.
60 Ibid., 300.
61 Jean Laplanche, quoted in Callard, "The Taming of Psychoanalysis," 304.
62 Freud, "The Ego and the Id (1923)," 397–8.
63 Thomas, "The Implications of Psychoanalysis," 537.
64 Ibid., 543.
65 Ibid.
66 Oliver, *The Colonization of Psychic Space*, xxii.
67 Shostak, *Interviewing and Representation*, 141.
68 Ibid.
69 Ibid., 72.
70 Ibid., 172.
71 Ibid., 173.
72 Ibid., 174.
73 Ibid.
74 Ibid., 175.
75 Ibid.
76 Holstein and Gubrium, *Inside Interviewing*, 20.
77 Ibid.
78 Richardson, "Poetic Representations of Interviews."
79 Rapport, "The Poetry of Holocaust Survivor Testimony."
80 Glesne, "'That Rare Feeling,'" 202–21.
81 Glesne, *Becoming Qualitative Researchers*, 183.
82 Ibid.
83 Ibid., 183.
84 Glesne "'That Rare Feeling,'" 215.
85 Glesne, *Becoming Qualitative Researchers*, 180.
86 Glesne, "'That Rare Feeling,'" 214.
87 Glesne, *Becoming Qualitative Researchers*, 178.
88 Glaser and Strauss, *The Discovery of Grounded Theory*, 101–16.

89 Glesne, *Becoming Qualitative Researchers*, 183.

90 Ibid., 187.

91 Paraphrased from Glesne, "'That Rare Feeling,'" 205.

92 Gilman, *Making the Body Beautiful*, 4. Gilman places the beginnings of modern cosmetic surgery around the 1880s and 1890s.

93 This notion is elaborated extensively in Gilman's *Creating Beauty to Cure the Soul*. While presently there is a great divide theoretically and clinically between psychology and psychoanalysis, during the foundational years of cosmetic surgery in the late nineteenth and early twentieth centuries, this divide was not so distinct. Psychology is the positivist study of human and animal mind and behaviour using the principles of the scientific method, whereas psychoanalysis is a theory and method developed by Sigmund Freud that is founded upon the notion of the unconscious and the importance of early childhood experiences for one's psychosexual development.

94 In particular, those differences coded as racial, ethnic, as well as extraordinary bodily configurations.

95 And indeed, with the exception of one interviewee (Nicanor), the interviewees are white women negotiating their understandings of femininity and women's bodies against this narrow model. See the appendix for more general information on the interviewees, including pseudonym, type of cosmetic surgery obtained, ethnicity/race, and age. Interviewees self-identified and filled out this information voluntarily at the time of the interview.

CHAPTER TWO

1 I elaborate on the connection between cosmetic surgery, classical aesthetics, and Western art later in this chapter when discussing the narratives of the cosmetic surgeon as artist and scientist.

2 I am not making a chronological argument here. Rather, I think that these shifts mark changes in attitudes toward cosmetic surgery and they occur repeatedly and cyclically in different places, at different times.

3 The cosmetic surgery story as a makeover story overcomes and encounters loss both in the sense that cosmetic surgery patients might seek out surgery as a response to a loss (of youth, former bodily configuration, or relationship, for example), just as the patient may also be confronted with loss by streamlining her story to make it appropriate to the surgeon and others, as well as the loss of the de-idealized body part.

4 Blum, *Flesh Wounds*, 126.

5 Gilman, *Making the Body Beautiful*, 10.

6 Ibid.

7 Davis, *Reshaping the Female Body*, 15.
8 Gilman, *Making the Body Beautiful*, 10.
9 Ibid.
10 Haiken, *Venus Envy*, 21.
11 Davis, *Reshaping the Female Body*, 15.
12 Gilman, *Making the Body Beautiful*, xxi.
13 Haiken, *Venus Envy*, 20–1.
14 Gilman, *Making the Body Beautiful*, xxi.
15 Ibid., 85.
16 Davis, *Dubious Equalities and Embodied Differences*, 90.
17 See Gilman, *Making the Body Beautiful*, 89–91.
18 Ibid., 91–8.
19 Ibid., 98–111.
20 Ibid., 111–18.
21 Davis, *Reshaping the Female Body*, 15.
22 Gilman, *Making the Body Beautiful*, 16.
23 Davis, *Reshaping the Female Body*, 15.
24 While one might be inclined at present to take for granted that the psychical (pertaining to the matters of the mind, including rational and psychological processes) and somatic (pertaining to the matters of the body, including all its physiological and biological processes) are deeply interconnected, the troubling and blurring of this distinction was a critical development for both psychoanalysis and cosmetic surgery.
25 The masculine pronoun is used intentionally here; men have historically been at the forefront of the development of cosmetic surgery, with the significant exception of Madame Suzanne Noël, who practised cosmetic surgery in the early twentieth century and developed face-lifting techniques, as well as materials that demystified cosmetic surgery for laypersons. For more on Noël, see Davis, "Cosmetic Surgery in a Different Voice," in *Dubious Equalities and Embodied Differences*, 19–39.
26 Gilman, *Making the Body Beautiful*, 12.
27 Haiken, *Venus Envy*, 110–11.
28 Gilman, *Making the Body Beautiful*, 309.
29 Gilman, *Creating Beauty to Cure the Soul*, xi.
30 The Hippocratic Oath in fact says no such thing, although it does dictate that doctors act only in the interests of curing the patient.
31 Blum, *Flesh Wounds*, 55.
32 Gilman, *Creating Beauty to Cure the Soul*, 12.
33 Stepansky, *Freud, Surgery, and the Surgeons*, 17.
34 Ibid., 18.
35 Ibid., 19.
36 Ibid., 20.

37 Gilman, *Creating Beauty to Cure the Soul*, 17.
38 Ibid., 14.
39 Ibid., 5.
40 Ibid., 142. Of course, this brings up the further conundrum that the features deemed anomalous shift across time and culture.
41 Otoplasty on children (commonly known as "ear pinning") is a good example of such a practice. While otoplasty was once considered a "cosmetic" surgery, it is now considered to be "reconstructive"; in Ontario, this means that it is covered by OHIP for children under eighteen years of age.
42 Gilman, *Creating Beauty to Cure the Soul*, 85. Freud was engaged in his self-analysis at the time.
43 Masson, *The Complete Letters*, 116–17.
44 Gilman, *Creating Beauty to Cure the Soul*, 93.
45 Menninger, "Polysurgery and Polysurgical Addiction," 175.
46 Gilman, *Creating Beauty to Cure the Soul*, 121.
47 Menninger, "Polysurgery and Polysurgical Addiction," 175.
48 Schilder, *Image and Appearance of the Human Body*, 15–16.
49 Gilman, *Creating Beauty to Cure the Soul*, 118–19.
50 Note that Adler did not use the term "inferiority complex," but the popular press attributed it to him because of his discussion of "inferiority" and a general American interest in Freud's and Jung's ideas of "complexes." For more on this, see Haiken, *Venus Envy*, 112.
51 Gilman, *Creating Beauty to Cure the Soul*, 101.
52 Haiken, *Venus Envy*, 118–19.
53 Davis, *Dubious Equalities and Embodied Differences*, 25.
54 Haiken, *Venus Envy*, 33.
55 Davis, *Dubious Equalities and Embodied Differences*, 43.
56 Haiken, *Venus Envy*, 50. We can see the strong desire on the part of cosmetic surgeons to delimit the profession of cosmetic surgery currently in the November 2007 statement that the Canadian Medical Association is planning to "crack down" on untrained practitioners of cosmetic surgery in response to a recent liposuction death in the Greater Toronto Area.
57 Gilman, *Making the Body Beautiful*, 164.
58 Haiken, *Venus Envy*, 133.
59 Ibid., 138.
60 Ibid., 135.
61 Ibid.
62 Ibid., 134.
63 Davis, *Dubious Equalities and Embodied Differences*, 89.
64 Haiken, *Venus Envy*, 132.
65 I return to this point in my description and analysis of the interviews I conducted with women who have undergone cosmetic surgery.

66 Haiken, *Venus Envy*, 149.

67 Davis, *Dubious Equalities and Embodied Differences*, 124 and 155.

68 Haiken, *Venus Envy*, 167–8.

69 Ibid., 175.

70 Davis, *Reshaping the Female Body*, 20.

71 Most recently, in 2005 Health Canada conducted a review of silicone breast implants to assess the possibility of re-licencing their sale by consulting communities of scientists, experts, and the public. (Prior to 2005, surgeons who wished to use silicone implants had to apply to Health Canada for permission.) As a result, Inamed, the manufacturer of silicone-filled breast implants, and Mentor, the manufacturer of cohesive silicone gel implants, were both granted licences to sell silicone breast implants in October 2006. See Health Canada, "Breast Implants."

72 Davis, *Reshaping the Female Body*, 30.

73 Ibid., 32. Davis's research on cosmetic surgery was done in the Netherlands at a time when the majority of cosmetic surgeries were funded by state health care.

74 Ibid., 32.

75 There are some exceptions to this case: in Canada, for example, the majority of breast reductions (which frequently include mastoplexy, or breast lifting, as well) are covered under provincial health insurance, as are some breast augmentations when a breast is removed.

76 For example, both an orthopaedic surgeon and a plastic surgeon would be able to perform hand surgery, or an otolaryngologist and a plastic surgeon could perform nose surgery.

77 Sullivan, *Cosmetic Surgery*, 78.

78 Ibid.

79 Frank, "Emily's Scars," 71. For example, a surgeon would use only a particular silicone implant manufactured by a corporation. In addition, many procedures are trademarked: Designer Laser Vaginoplasty™, for instance.

80 Blum, *Flesh Wounds*, 4.

81 It is important to note here that this gaze of the surgeon is one that is imagined and often constructed through representations of cosmetic surgeons in popular media. Just as patients have a diverse range of attitudes and reasons for their involvement with the cosmetic surgery industry, so too do cosmetic surgeons. While the imagined gaze may correspond to the individual surgeon's gaze, this is not necessarily the case.

82 Zong and Tsentserensky, "Services" and "Footcare Dictionary."

83 Matlock, "The Laser Vaginal Rejuvenation Institute of Los Angeles."

84 Ibid.

85 American Orthopaedic Foot and Ankle Society, "Cosmetic Foot Surgery."

86 Laliberté, "New Vaginas for Old."
87 Blum, *Flesh Wounds*, 38.
88 Ibid., 33.
89 Ibid., 32.
90 Martin, "Suffering for Beauty," 54.
91 Gerstel, "Breast Implants with Own Flesh," E2.
92 Gooden, "The Changing Face of Cosmetic Surgery," 58.
93 Kazanjian, "The Wrinkles We Keep," 196.
94 Ibid.
95 Gooden and Gee, "The Made-to-order Face," 81.
96 Wong, "A Closer Look at the Double-fold Dream," M3.
97 Benjamin, "10 Shocking Truths," 200.
98 Gearey, "Size Does Matter," F7.
99 Hall, "'Ethnic Surgery' on Rise," E4.
100 Mahoney, "Designer Vaginas," A1.
101 Blum, *Flesh Wounds*, 93.
102 Matlock, "The Laser Vaginal Rejuvenation Institute of Los Angeles."
103 Ibid.
104 Davis, "Loose Lips Sink Ships," 27.
105 For examples, see Blum, *Flesh Wounds*, 14, and Davis, *Reshaping the Female Body*, 37.
106 Etcoff, *Survival of the Prettiest*, 25.
107 Ibid., 9.
108 Stacey, "Are Butts the New Boobs?," 154–7.
109 Izzo, "Afraid to Show Your Hand?" L1.
110 Zong, "The Pinky Toe Tuck."
111 Zong, "NYCFootcare."
112 Ibid.
113 Ibid.
114 Ford and Mitchell, *The Makeover in Movies*, 63.
115 Ibid., 132.
116 Ibid., 16.
117 Davis, *Reshaping the Female Body*, 97.
118 Ibid.
119 Ibid., 97–8.
120 Ibid., 98.
121 Blum, *Flesh Wounds*, 23.
122 Blum, *Flesh Wounds*, 17. In one of her interviews with cosmetic surgeons, Blum was asked this very question and later concludes that this question is central to women's identity.
123 My Google search of "double eyelid fold surgery" yielded multiple examples. The first surgeon's website listed in the search results was a good one: Lee, "Asian Eyelid Surgery."
124 Davis, *Reshaping the Female Body*, 91.
125 Blum, *Flesh Wounds*, 76.

126 Ibid., 290.
127 Deery, "Interior Design," 169.
128 Jerslev, "The Mediated Body," 136.
129 Ouellette and Hay, *Better Living through Reality TV*, 3.
130 Ibid., 7.
131 Deery, "Interior Design," 170.
132 Jerslev, "The Mediated Body," 142.
133 Ouellette and Hay, *Better Living through Reality TV*, 102.
134 If indeed we can say that legitimate psychological work was done at all! The life coach, Nely Galan, is also the producer of the show, which throws the motivations and qualifications of all others involved in the show into question.
135 Blum, *Flesh Wounds*, 109.
136 Eastlake, quoted in Di Bello, "The 'Eyes of Affection' and Fashionable Femininity," 257.
137 The photograph is essential for cosmetic surgery, a point to which I return in chapter 3. However, since I have just discussed a *television* makeover show, it seems useful to reflect briefly on the differences between photography and moving images like television and film. While the moving image that does not reflect how we imagine our bodies may be just as alienating as the photograph, it does not allow us to fixate on our features in the same way precisely because the image moves. And, as I discuss in greater detail later in this chapter, the stillness of the photograph, which imitates the stillness of death, enables the fantasy of cosmetic surgery because it is psychically easier to distance that fantasy from the corporeal reality of cutting, burning, and removal of flesh. Cosmetic surgery reality television shows use photographs as evidence of the transformative result, and sometimes the photograph is manipulated pre-surgery to demonstrate the benefits of the surgery. For example, *The Swan* uses a photographic three-dimensional representation that stays still, rotates, or floats on a grid-like background to identify the "problem" areas that can be addressed through surgery. Instantly, the floating digital representation doubles, and is altered digitally. The final beauty pageant features before and after photographs to demonstrate how the contestants have changed. I suggest that the television show that focuses on cosmetic surgery is not able to effectively show transformation through the moving image, and remains reliant on the photograph to do this work. As an aside, other makeover shows that transform rooms, gardens, and cars also often use a montage of photographic images to show transformation, even though these objects do not move themselves.
138 Adams, quoted in Prosser, *Second Skins*, 208.
139 Metz, quoted in Grant, "Still Moving Images," 66.
140 Prosser, *Second Skins*, n.p.
141 Barthes, *Camera Lucida*, 9.

142 Ibid., 14.
143 Sontag, *On Photography*, 154.
144 Durand, quoted in Lury, *Prosthetic Culture*, 149.
145 Lury, *Prosthetic Culture*, 149.
146 Prosser, *Light in the Dark Room*, 2.
147 Benjamin, "The Work of Art in the Age of Mechanical Reproduction," 226.
148 Ibid.
149 Sontag, *On Photography*, 80.
150 Barthes, *Camera Lucida*, 34.
151 Ibid.
152 Freud, *The Uncanny*, 143.
153 Ibid., 148.
154 Lacan, *The Four Fundamental Concepts*, 106.
155 Prosser, *Light in the Dark Room*, 7.
156 Ibid., 10.
157 Ibid., 7.
158 Davidov, "Narratives of Place," 41.
159 Barthes, *Camera Lucida*, 15 (grammatical error in text).
160 Ibid., 80–1.
161 Davis, *Reshaping the Female Body*, 70.
162 Barthes, *Camera Lucida*, 103.
163 Benjamin, "The Work of Art in the Age of Mechanical Reproduction," 220.
164 Sontag, *On Photography*, 110.
165 Siegel, "Talking through the 'Fotygraft Album,'" 241.
166 Lury, *Prosthetic Culture*, 84.
167 Prosser, *Light in the Dark Room*, 10–11.
168 Benjamin, "The Work of Art in the Age of Mechanical Reproduction," 233–4.
169 Ibid, 233.
170 Ibid., 233–4.
171 Ibid., 234.
172 Ibid., 236.
173 Ibid., 237.
174 Sontag, *On Photography*, 85.
175 Ibid., 3.
176 Ibid., 4.
177 Blum, *Flesh Wounds*, 199.
178 Ibid., 198.
179 Ibid., 199.
180 Ibid., 203.
181 Rogers, "The First Pre- and Post-Operative Photographs of Plastic and Reconstructive Surgery," 21.
182 Rogers and Rhond, "The First Civil War Photographs," 270.

183 Gilman, *Making the Body Beautiful*, 38.
184 Meyerowitz, "Beyond the Feminine Mystique," 233.

CHAPTER THREE

1 Blum, *Flesh Wounds*, 200.
2 All that I describe here constitutes what Barthes calls the *studium* of the photograph, or a general examination of the details of the photograph that would be agreed upon by most who look at it, while I only allude to the *punctum*, or the "small hole" in the photograph, that represents a point of the photograph that pierces me (the gap-toothed smile on my shadowed face) and is particular and important only to me. See Barthes, *Camera Lucida*, 25–8 for more on the *studium* and *punctum*.
3 Connor, *The Book of Skin*, 59.
4 Ibid.
5 Ibid.
6 The use of photography in the specific practice of cosmetic surgery exists among the general use of photography in surface imagination cultures to construct and narrate identity as evidenced by the proliferation of technologies to capture images (like camera phones and digital cameras) and forums or opportunities to disseminate images (such as text messaging and the Internet). These hold the image to be the definitive expression of the self, an object that can attain a perfection that the body is incapable of achieving and through which we can narrate who we are to others.
7 I elaborate these ideas later in this chapter through the work of Silverman.
8 Billie and Sørenson, "An Anthropology of Luminosity," 266.
9 Berger, *Ways of Seeing*, 17.
10 Ibid., 46.
11 I assume that Tonya was referring to "phantom limb syndrome," which describes the phenomenon of continuing to feel sensations in a limb that has been amputated.
12 I should note here that Victoria's chemical peels and laser treatments do not carry the same risks of death through adverse reactions to anaesthesia or development of sepsis that the other six interviewees faced. See my footnoted discussion about the relationship between Victoria's procedures and cosmetic surgery in the second chapter, which also includes a discussion of the differences between Victoria's procedures and the procedures of the other interviewees.
13 Silverman, *The Threshold of the Visible World*, 11.
14 Ibid.
15 Ibid., 12.

16 Ibid., 13.

17 Ibid., 14.

18 Ibid.

19 Lacan, "The Mirror Stage," 1–2.

20 Silverman, *The Threshold of the Visible World*, 15.

21 Ibid.

22 Ibid., 16.

23 However, there are some exceptions: conspiracy theorists are very interested in the way that police and military photographs have been doctored to conceal evidence.

24 This is a perception formed from having four friends and acquaintances who underwent the procedure, as well as being a person with "disproportionately" large breasts that would likely be eligible for insurance coverage for this surgery in Ontario. Diane Naugler's dissertation contains several narratives that corroborate this perception as well. See Naugler, "To Take a Load Off."

25 When Diana and I met, her three-month follow up appointment was scheduled for later in the week. Diana wasn't sure if her surgeon would take photographs at that appointment, but thought that it was likely.

26 I should note here that Tonya did not indicate one way or another if she would have proceeded with the breast reduction if it hadn't been approved for coverage. Leah, on the other hand, indicated strongly that she would have had the breast reduction "no matter what."

27 Of course, the determination of whether the patient's claim is justified or not is first made by the surgeon.

28 This is more likely in the United States than in Canada, because of the United States' private health care system and relative ease of filing lawsuits against those in the medical profession.

29 My provincial driver's license from 1994 bears a black and white photograph, and my passport of the same year also has a black and white photograph. I recently reapplied for a passport, and now it is acceptable to submit either a colour or a black and white photograph.

30 Indeed, on many surgeons' websites, usually only the age, sex, procedures, and length of time between the procedure and photograph accompany the images. One interesting exception is breast augmentation, which frequently also includes the cup sizes of the women's breasts before and after, as well as the number of CCs (cubic centimetres) of saline or silicone contained in the implant.

31 This has since changed. In 2006, Health Canada re-approved the use of silicone implants.

32 Even though she had numbness on the side of her face that bothered her, Tigerlily expressed very definitely that her surgery was not that bad in terms of suffering.

33 I did this because I was interested in seeing them, and because I thought they might be useful cues or props for Tigerlily to construct her narrative. However, she was unable to find them; she did not know what happened to the photographs she took after her surgery.

34 Silverman, *The Threshold of the Visible World*, 33 (her emphasis). Note that the "negative" resolution of the Oedipal complex for the girl refers to continuing to take the mother as love object and identifying with the father, in contrast to the "positive" resolution of the Oedipal complex, where the girl shifts her love to her father and chooses instead to identify with her mother. The latter is referred to as "normal" femininity in Freud, and the former is the masculinity complex.

35 Ibid.

36 Ibid.

37 Ibid., 34.

38 Ibid.

39 Freud, quoted in Silverman, *The Threshold of the Visible World*, 34.

40 Silverman, *The Threshold of the Visible World*, 37.

41 Lacan, *The Seminar of Jacques Lacan, Book VII: The Ethics of Psychoanalysis*, 99.

42 Silverman, *The Threshold of the Visible World*, 80–1.

43 Ibid., 19.

44 Ibid., 20.

45 Ibid., 29.

46 ORLAN is an exemplary figure as she "queers" cosmetic surgery *and* is mindful of the social and economic contexts that her work is queering. As a result, her work is particularly salient when read in relation to the narratives of "ordinary" women who undergo cosmetic surgery. See, for example, Davis's discussion of these connections in her chapter "'My Body is My Art,'" in *Dubious Equalities*, 105–16. While the topic of queering cosmetic surgery through art and experimental surgical practice is intriguing, it dovetails less well with the narratives in this book. In my reading of such endeavours, this utopic or hypothetical engagement is less relevant to the ordinary experiences of cosmetic surgery because it often elides an engagement with the social and economic conditions that structure cosmetic surgery as a cultural practice. For excellent analyses that read this social and economic context into these practices, see the work of Meredith Jones, particularly in her discussions of surgeons like Joe Rosen in *Skintight* and adult celebrity Lolo Ferrari in "Makeover Culture's Dark Side."

47 Phelan, "Cinematic Skin," 73.

48 O'Bryan, *Carnal Art*, xi.

49 Ince, ORLAN: *Millennial Female*, 131.

50 Ibid.
51 Adams, *The Emptiness of the Image*, 159.
52 Ibid.
53 Ibid., 143–4.
54 Adams discusses at length ORLAN's assertion that she is a "woman to woman transsexual" (144), an intriguing claim, but one that I fear would sidetrack my focus on photography here. In the following chapter, I explore this conceptualization of the "wrong body" in transsexual narratives through the work of Nikki Sullivan.
55 Ibid., 144.
56 Ibid., 145.
57 Ibid.
58 Ibid., 159.
59 Ibid.

CHAPTER FOUR

1 Connor, *The Book of Skin*, 90.
2 The unintentional cut, bruise, and scar inscribed into the skin are examples of how we experience contingency and accident through the skin, a subject I explore in this chapter. These skin-experiences remind us that our skins are not invulnerable and that the external world is unpredictable and may inscribe its mark on us at any time.
3 See Prosser, *Second Skins*, and Connor, *The Book of Skin*. While my use of the phrase "second skin" is informed by both Prosser and Connor, I tend use it more colloquially in this chapter and rely more heavily on Connor's conceptualization, making the distinctions when necessary through referencing and explanation. Prosser uses the phrase "second skin" in two ways: first, to describe the way that clothing may hold transsexual bodies and provide an external casing (Prosser, *Second Skins*, 75); and second, he describes narrative as a second skin that clothes transsexual bodies by legitimizing transition for the self and others (ibid., 112). Prosser's conceptualization of the "second skin" is deeply influenced by Anzieu's metaphor of the skin ego, and particularly the holding function of the skin as it develops through the mother-baby bond. Connor, on the other hand, emphasizes doubling in his conceptualization of the "second skin," focusing on the figures of the stigmatic and the hysteric in his discussion (Connor, *The Book of Skin*, 135–42). What I like about Connor's formulation of the "second skin" is its insistence on the inseparability of the psychical and physical skin, a significant component of the "doubling" he discusses. My concern about Prosser's interpretation of the "second skin" is that he sometimes privileges what he calls "materiality" of the skin over the psychical elements of skin. For an excellent

critique of these tendencies in Prosser's *Second Skins*, see Elliot, "A Psychoanalytic Reading of Transsexual Embodiment."

4 Freud, "The Ego and the Id" (1923), 398.

5 Ibid., 397–8.

6 Freud, "The Unconscious" (1915), 172.

7 Ibid., 191.

8 Freud "The Ego and the Id" (1923), 364, his emphasis.

9 Ibid.

10 Ibid.

11 Freud, "A Note on the Mystic Writing-Pad" (1925), 430.

12 Anzieu, *The Skin Ego*, 10.

13 Nanomaterial Science Lab, "Skin Structure."

14 Anzieu, *The Skin Ego*, 4.

15 Ibid., 6.

16 Ibid.

17 Ibid., 7.

18 Ibid., 8–9.

19 Ibid., 40.

20 Ibid.

21 Here I am adhering to Anzieu's decision to use "phantasy" over "fantasy," a decision that implies an alliance with ego psychology and the British object relations school of psychoanalytic theory.

22 Anzieu, *The Skin Ego*, 4.

23 Ibid., 97.

24 Ibid., 61.

25 Ibid.

26 Ibid.

27 Ibid.

28 Ibid., 84.

29 Ibid., 175.

30 Ibid., 40.

31 Ibid.

32 Ibid., 39–40.

33 This is narcissism "in the regular course of human sexual development," according to Freud in "On Narcissism (1914)," 65–6.

34 Anzieu, *The Skin Ego*, 41.

35 Ibid., 231.

36 For more on skin as a textile in cosmetic surgery, see my chapter "The Skin-Textile in Cosmetic Surgery," 141–66.

37 Connor, *The Book of Skin*, 82.

38 Ibid., 79.

39 Ibid., 73.

40 Ibid., 90.

41 A line of inquiry that intrigued me, but that I eventually chose not to

follow, was the function of shame in cosmetic surgery narratives. I was delighted, therefore, when Jane Megan Northrop's book *Reflecting on Cosmetic Surgery* was published in 2012. Northrop examines shame in cosmetic surgery narratives, and argues that the normalization of narcissism has emerged as a way of correcting embodied shame.

42 Biven, "The Role of Skin," 223.

43 Connor, *The Book of Skin*, 64.

44 Ibid., 54.

45 Ibid., 56.

46 These are just a few examples of skin transformations that I identified as related to cosmetic surgery. Of course, there are many others: tattooing, scarification, piercing, to name a few.

47 In the recording, while I think it is most likely that Leah was saying "ooh and ah," it is also possible that she said, "*ew* and ah." Within the context of her other comments about her post-surgical body, I do not think that a selection of one over the other compromises the meaning.

48 The hidden and visible scars in cosmetic surgery have more in common than we might initially think. Both mark a moment in time in which a second skin is formed. The visible scar is a mark that tells of controlling time and is a sign of that control that can be perceived by the self and others. The hidden scar is a mark that tells of concealing time, and is a sign of control that is perceived only by the self and those in the know (the scar's wearer controls this access).

49 For more on beauty and skin colour, see Seshadri-Crooks, *Desiring Whiteness*; McClintock, *Imperial Leather*; and Hunter, *Race, Gender and the Politics of Skin Tone*, particularly her chapter "Black and Brown Bodies under the Knife," 53–67.

50 Connor, *The Book of Skin*, 90.

51 Ibid., 74.

52 Ibid., 90.

53 Ibid., 74.

54 Ibid., 52.

55 Ibid., 51.

56 Ibid., 52.

57 While not directly related to my discussion of the scar in cosmetic surgery, there is a fairly large body of literature that explores the role of the scar and the cut in body modification practices such as scarification, the tattoo, piercing, and suspension. For some recent examples, see Pitts, *In the Flesh*; Burr and Hearn, *Sex, Violence, and the Body*; and Williams, *Self-Mutilation*. Scarry's discussion of the un-making and re-making of the body in pain is also an interesting way of examining the cut and scar in cosmetic surgery, although it is outside of the scope of this book. See Scarry, *The Body in Pain*.

58 Benthien, *Skin*, 1.

59 Prosser, *Second Skins*, 62.

60 Benthien, *Skin*, 24.

61 Ibid., 27–8. Note that in my paraphrasing of Benthien's list, I have chosen not to discuss the body-house or the body, but have altered this to refer specifically to the skin.

62 Anonymous surgeon, quoted in Blum, *Flesh Wounds*, 76.

63 I say "so-called physical experience of the body and transition" here because Prosser tends to reduce the bodily ego to its supposedly physical manifestations and minimizes the psychical aspects of the body ego through an emphasis on the supposedly biological and social aspects of the body. Once again, Elliot's article offers a good analysis of Prosser's insistence on the "materiality" of the body.

64 Prosser, *Second Skins*, 68–9.

65 Ibid., 73.

66 Anzieu, *The Skin Ego*, 51.

67 Prosser, *Second Skins*, 73.

68 Of course, there are many ways that we accept this misfortune aside from surgeries.

69 Prosser, *Second Skins*, 71.

70 Anzieu, *The Skin Ego*, 20.

71 In this digression, I focus on non-genital sex reassignment surgeries whose primary goal is to change the appearance of the body: for example, breast augmentation, bilateral mastectomy, chest reconstruction, facial feminization surgery, tracheal shaving, and facial feminization surgery. Of course, genital sex reassignment surgeries also alter the appearance of the body, but they have less in common with surgeries that non-transsexual people seek that are termed "cosmetic." I also use "transsexual" in this section to refer to individuals who seek out surgery and hormones to facilitate transition from one sex to another, with full awareness of the limitations of this definition. This is the terminology most commonly used by medical professionals and health insurance documents, which is why I have made this decision.

72 It is important to note here that this is the dominant and acceptable discourse about seeking cosmetic surgery; I discuss the tension between the notion that cosmetic surgery is an individual decision made in isolation and the reality that cosmetic surgery is a decision that is made in *relation* to others in my article "Negotiating Femininity."

73 For more detail, see OHIP, "Schedule of Benefits."

74 While other sex reassignment surgeries for transsexual individuals are covered by OHIP, breast augmentation is not.

75 I mention transability here as an experience of embodiment that relies on the narrative of the "wrong body," which has more recently come

to the attention of critical disability and trans studies, and pushes the boundaries of both. For more on transability, see Baril and Trevenen, "Exploring Ableism and Cisnormativity" and Baril's "Needing to Acquire a Physical Impairment/Disability." In "The Role of Medicine," Nikki Sullivan focuses on what she terms "self-demand amputees" or "wannabes," which Baril clarifies ought to be understood as part of the transabled umbrella, but not its entirety.

76 Prosser, *Second Skins*, 70; and Sullivan, "The Role of Medicine," 105. Sullivan's article is concerned with making connections between transsexual and transabled narratives, although she uses the terminology of "self-demand amputees" and "wannabes."

77 Sullivan, "The Role of Medicine," 107.

78 Ibid., 108–10.

79 Sullivan gives the example of Christine Jorgensen, who was first diagnosed as homosexual and received treatment under that premise, not that she was a transsexual woman. She also notes that individual practitioners undoubtedly had other motives and sought to alleviate the suffering of their patients; however, the point is that the official motivations were deeply conservative. Ibid., 109.

80 Ibid., 112.

81 Ibid.

82 Heyes, *Self-Transformations*, 119.

83 Ibid.

84 Of course, ideals and norms of masculinity similarly structure men's encounters with cosmetic surgery, whether they are trans or not. The point here is that the ambiguously gendered body is never positioned as desirable within the ideology of cosmetic surgery.

85 Which is not to say that none of them were trans identified!

86 Lemma, "The Body One Has and the Body One Is," 278–9.

87 Ibid., 278.

88 Winncott, quoted in Lemma, "The Body One Has and the Body One Is," 278.

89 Lemma, "The Body One Has and the Body One Is," 278–9.

90 Ibid., 285.

91 Ibid., 284.

92 Ibid., 285.

93 Winnicott, quoted in Lemma, "The Body One Has and the Body One Is," 278.

94 Salecl, "Cut in the Body," 21.

95 It is important to note here that Salecl is not claiming that clitoridectomy is the *same* as other "cutting" body modification practices like cosmetic surgery. Rather, she is attempting to theorize the coincidence of a range of "cutting" body modification practices within postmodern society. The example of clitoridectomy is included here to demonstrate

the effects of such a reconceptualization, before moving into Salecl's other example of body art in the global North, which resonates more with cosmetic surgery.

96 Van Pelt, *The Other Side of Desire*, 48.
97 Lacan, *The Psychoses*, 9–10.
98 Van Pelt, *The Other Side of Desire*, 52.
99 Ibid., 49.
100 Ibid., 53.
101 Ibid., 51.
102 Ibid., 137.
103 Ibid., 49.
104 Ibid., 69.
105 Ibid.
106 Ibid., 71.
107 Salecl, "Cut in the Body," 25.
108 Ibid., 27.
109 Ibid.
110 Ibid.
111 Ibid.
112 Ibid., 25.
113 Ibid.
114 Ibid.
115 Ibid.
116 Castration is an unfortunately gendered word used to explain a condition of lack that we all share, regardless of gender, that is instantiated in our entry into the symbolic through language acquisition.
117 Salecl, "Cut in the Body," 31.
118 Ibid., 32.

CONCLUSION

1 This conceptualization comes from Blum's lovely notion of the "body landscape." See Blum, *Flesh Wounds*, 41–4.
2 Illouz, *Cold Intimacies*, 4.
3 Ibid.
4 This is not just a distance between the speaker and the cosmetic surgery patient, but it is also an assumption that I am similarly distanced from the cosmetic surgery patient.
5 I will also note that this response originates from a privileged position of *not knowing* what it feels like to suffer so severely from one's appearance that surgery becomes a viable option.
6 Lemma, *Under the Skin*, 12.
7 Ibid.

8 In Canada, statistics are not kept for surgical or non-surgical cosmetic procedures. However, the American Society for Aesthetic Plastic Surgery reports that in 2011, over nine million surgical and non-surgical procedures were performed in the United States. See American Society for Aesthetic Plastic Surgery, "Quick Facts."

9 By "fix" I mean here both the sense of repairing the body and positioning it in a particular location and time.

10 Silverman, *The Threshold of the Visible World*, 2.

11 Britzman, *Lost Subjects, Contested Objects*, 41.

12 Silverman, *The Threshold of the Visible World*, 224.

13 Ibid.

14 Lemma, *Under the Skin*, 3.

15 These phantasies are traced throughout her book; the "reclaiming phantasy" is investigated in chapters 4, 5, and 8; the "perfect match phantasy" is investigated in chapters 1, 4, and 7; and the "self-made phantasy" is investigated in chapters 4, 6, 7, and 8.

16 Silverman, *The Threshold of the Visible World*, 227.

A NOTE ON THE COVER

1 Yeo, Personal website.

BIBLIOGRAPHY

Adams, Parveen. *The Emptiness of the Image: Psychoanalysis and Sexual Difference*. London and New York: Routledge, 1996

Allen, Robert. *Beauty Surgeon: Behind the Scenes with Hollywood's Famous Plastic Surgeon*. Long Beach, CA: Whitehorn, 1960

American Orthopedic Foot and Ankle Society. "Cosmetic Foot Surgery." http://www.aofas.org/i4a/pages/index.cfm?pageid=3672. Accessed 27 July 2007

American Society of Plastic Surgeons. "2011 Quick Facts." http://www.plasticsurgery.org/Documents/news-resources/statistics/2011-statistics/2011_Stats_Quick_Facts.pdf. Accessed 6 July 2012

Anzieu, Didier. *The Skin Ego*. Translated by Chris Turner. New Haven: Yale University Press, 1989

Armstrong, Rachel. "Anger, Art and Medicine: Working with Orlan." In *Cyborg Experiments: The Extensions of the Body in the Media Age*, edited by Joanna Zylinksa, 172–8. London: Continuum, 2002

Balsamo, Anne. "On the Cutting Edge: Cosmetic Surgery and the Technological Production of the Gendered Body." In Balsamo, *Technologies of the Gendered Body*, 207–37

– *Technologies of the Gendered Body: Reading Cyborg Women*. Durham: Duke University Press, 1996

Baril, Alexandre. "Needing to Acquire a Physical Impairment/Disability: (Re)Thinking the Connections between Trans and Disability Studies through Transability." Translated by Catriona LeBlanc. *Hypatia: Journal of Feminist Philosophy* 30, no. 1 (2014). Published online through Early View

Baril, Alexandre, and Kathryn Trevenen. "Exploring Ableism and Cisnormativity in the Conceptualization of Identity and Sexuality 'Disorders.'" *Annual Review of Critical Psychology* 11 (2014): 389–416

Barthes, Roland. *Camera Lucida: Reflections on Photography*. New York: Hill and Wang, 1981

Benjamin, Jennifer. "10 Shocking Truths about Plastic Surgery." *Cosmopolitan* 240, 2 (February 2006): 196–9

Benjamin, Walter. "The Work of Art in the Age of Mechanical Reproduction." In *Illuminations*, edited by Hannah Arendt, 217–51. New York: Schocken, 1968

Benthien, Claudia. *Skin: On the Cultural Border between Self and the World*. Translated by Thomas Dunlap. New York: Columbia University Press, 2003

Berger, John. *Ways of Seeing*. London: BBC and Penguin Books, 1972
Billie, Mikkel, and Tim Flohr Sørenson. "An Anthropology of Luminosity."
    Journal of Material Culture 12, no. 3 (2007): 263–84
Biven, Barrie M. "The Role of Skin in Normal and Abnormal Development
    with a Note on the Poet Sylvia Plath." *International Review of Psycho-
    Analysis* 63, no. 9 (1982): 205–29
Blair, Vilray Papin. "Underdeveloped Jaw, with Limited Excursion." *Jour-
    nal of the American Medical Association* 53, no. 3 (1909): 178–83
Blum, Virginia. *Flesh Wounds: The Culture of Cosmetic Surgery*. Berkeley:
    University of California Press, 2003
Bordo, Susan. "Material Girl: The Effacements of Postmodern Culture."
    In *The Gender/Sexuality Reader: Culture, History, Political Economy*,
    edited by Roger Lancaster and Micaela de Leonardo, 653–77. London:
    Routledge 1997
Bourdieu, Pierre. *In Other Words: Essays towards a Reflexive Sociology*.
    Cambridge: Polity Press, 1990
Britzman, Deborah P. *Lost Subjects, Contested Objects: Toward a Psycho-
    analytic Inquiry of Learning*. Albany: State University of New York
    Press, 1998
Burr, Viv, and Jeff Hearn, editors. *Sex, Violence, and the Body: The Erotics
    of Wounding*. New York: Palgrave, 2008
Callard, Felicity. "The Taming of Psychoanalysis in Geography." *Social &
    Cultural Geography* 4, no. 3 (2003): 295–312
Charmaz, Kathy. *Constructing Grounded Theory: A Practical Guide through
    Qualitative Analysis*. Thousand Oaks, CA: SAGE Publications, 2006
Cheng, Anne Anlin. *Second Skin: Josephine Baker and the Modern Surface*.
    Oxford: Oxford University Press, 2011
Clarke, Adele E. *Situational Analysis: Grounded Theory after the Postmod-
    ern Turn*. Thousand Oaks, CA: SAGE Publications, 2005
Connor, Steven. *The Book of Skin*. Ithaca: Cornell University Press, 2004
Covino, Deborah Caslav. *Amending the Abject Body: Aesthetic Makeovers
    in Medicine and Culture*. Albany: SUNY Press, 2004
Davidov, Judith Fryer. "Narratives of Place: History and Memory in the
    Evidential Force of Photography in Work by Meridel Rubenstein and
    Joan Myers." In Hughes and Noble, *Phototextualities*, 41–63
Davis, Kathy. *Dubious Equalities and Embodied Differences: Cultural
    Studies on Cosmetic Surgery*. Lanham: Rowman and Littlefield, 2003
– *Reshaping the Female Body: The Dilemma of Cosmetic Surgery*. New
    York and London: Routledge, 1995
Davis, Simone Weil. "Loose Lips Sink Ships." *Feminist Studies* 28, no. 1
    (Spring 2002): 7–35
Deery, June. "Interior Design: Commodifying Self and Place in *Extreme
    Makeover, Extreme Makeover: Home Edition*, and *The Swan*." In *The*

Great American Makeover: Television, History, Nation, edited by Dana Heller, 159–74. New York: Palgrave, 2006

Di Bello, Patrizia. "The 'Eyes of Affection' and Fashionable Femininity: Representations of Photography in Nineteenth-Century Magazines and Victorian 'Society' Albums." In *Phototextualities: Intersections of Photography and Narrative,* edited by Alex Hughes and Andrea Noble, 254–70. Albuquerque: University of New Mexico Press, 2003

Dowling, N., A.C. Jackson, R.J. Honigman, and K.L. Francis. "Psychological Characteristics and Outcomes of Elective Cosmetic Surgery Patients: The Influence of Cosmetic Surgery History." *Plastic Surgical Nursing* 31, no. 4 (2011): 176–84

Edmond, Alexander. *Pretty Modern: Beauty, Sex, and Plastic Surgery in Brazil.* Durham: Duke University Press, 2010

Elliott, Patricia. "A Psychoanalytic Reading of Transsexual Embodiment." *Studies in Gender and Sexuality* 2, no. 4 (2001): 295–325

Etcoff, Nancy. *Survival of the Prettiest: The Science of Beauty.* New York: Doubleday, 1999

"Facelift Photos: iEnhance Photo Gallery." http://www.ienhance.com/ physician/page3_case_description.asp?DocID=57203&ProcImageID= 14883. Accessed 30 January 2008

Felman, Shoshana. *What Does a Woman Want? Reading and Sexual Difference.* Baltimore: Johns Hopkins University Press, 1993

Ford, Elizabeth A., and Deborah C. Mitchell. *The Makeover in Movies: Before and After in Hollywood Films, 1941–2002.* Jefferson, NC and London: McFarland & Company, 2004

Frank, Arthur W. "Emily's Scars: Surgical Shapings, Technoluxe, and Bioethics." In *Surgically Shaping Children: Technology, Ethics, and the Pursuit of Normativity,* edited by Erik Parens, 68–89. Baltimore: Johns Hopkins University Press, 2006

Fraser, Suzanne. *Cosmetic Surgery, Gender and Culture.* Basingstoke: Palgrave, 2003

Freud, Sigmund. "The Dissection of the Psychical Personality (1933)." In *New Introductory Lectures on Psycho-Analysis,* translated by James Strachey, 57–80. London: Hogarth Press, 1955

– "The Ego and the Id" (1923). In *On Metapsychology,* translated by James Strachey, 350–407. New York: Penguin Books, 1984

– "On Narcissism" (1914). In *On Metapsychology,* translated by James Strachey, 427–34. New York: Penguin Books, 1984

– "A Note on the Mystic Writing-Pad" (1925). In *On Metapsychology,* translated by James Strachey, 428–34. New York: Penguin Books, 1984

– *The Uncanny.* New York: Penguin Books, 2003

– "The Unconscious" (1915). In *On Metapsychology,* translated by James Strachey, 167–222. New York: Penguin Books, 1984

Frueh, Joanna. *Swooning Beauty: A Memoir of Pleasure*. Reno: University of Nevada Press, 2005

Gearey, Jenn. "Size Does Matter: Jenn Gearey Explains Why, 10 Years after Having Her Breasts Reduced, She Changed Her Mind and Went under the Knife Again." *Globe and Mail* (2 December 2006), F7

Gerstel, Judy. "Breast Implants with Own Flesh; Liposuction Used to Supply Fat for Augmentation Toronto Surgeon Says Technique Best in Some Cases." *Toronto Star*, 11 August 2006, E2.

Gilman, Sander. *Creating Beauty to Cure the Soul: Race and Psychology in the Shaping of Aesthetic Surgery*. Durham: Duke University Press, 1998

– *Making the Body Beautiful: A Cultural History of Aesthetic Surgery*. Princeton: Princeton University Press, 1999

Gimlin, Debra. *Body Work: Beauty and Self-Image in American Culture*. Berkeley: University of California Press 2002

– *Cosmetic Surgery Narratives: A Cross-Cultural Analysis of Women's Accounts*. Basingstoke: Palgrave, 2012

Glaser, Barney G., and Anselm L. Strauss. *The Discovery of Grounded Theory: Strategies for Qualitative Research*. New York: Aldine, 1967

Glesne, Corrine. *Becoming Qualitative Researchers: An Introduction*, 2nd ed. New York: Longman, 1999

– "'That Rare Feeling': Re-presenting Research through Poetic Transcription." *Qualitative Inquiry* 3, no. 2 (1997): 202–21

Gooden, Charmaine. "The Changing Face of Cosmetic Surgery." *Chatelaine* 69, 3 (March 1996): 56–9

Gooden, Charmaine, and Miriam Gee. "The Made-to-order Face." *Chatelaine* 66, no. 4 (April 1993): 81

Grant, Catherine. "Still Moving Images: Photographs of the Disappeared in Films about the 'Dirty War' in Argentina." In Hughes and Noble, *Phototextualities*, 63–86

Gubrium, Jaber F., and James Holstein, editors. *Handbook of Interview Research*. London: SAGE Publications, 2002

Haiken, Elizabeth. *Venus Envy: A History of Cosmetic Surgery*. Baltimore: Johns Hopkins University Press, 1997

Hall, Joseph. "'Ethnic Surgery' on Rise, Doctors Say Patients Seeking Western Look with Nose, Eye Work." *Toronto Star*, 16 September 2006, E4

Harding, Sandra. *Sciences from Below: Feminisms, Postcolonialities, and Modernities*. Durham: Duke University Press, 2008

Health Canada. "Breast Implants: Licensing Decision on Silicone Gel-filled Breast Implants." http://www.hc-sc.gc.ca/dhp-mps/md-im/activit/sci-consult/implant-breast-mammaire/index_e.html. Accessed 24 July 2007

Heller, Dana, editor. *The Great American Makeover: Television, History, Nation*. New York: Palgrave, 2006

Heyes, Cressida. *Self-Transformations: Foucault, Ethics, and Normalized Bodies*. Oxford: Oxford University Press, 2007

Heyes, Cressida, and Meredith Jones, editors. *Cosmetic Surgery: A Feminist Primer*. Surrey: Ashgate, 2009

Holliday, Ruth, and Jacqueline Sanchez Taylor. "Aesthetic Surgery as False Beauty." *Feminist Theory* 7, no. 2 (2006): 179–95

Holstein, James, and Jaber F. Gubrium, editors. *Inside Interviewing: New Lenses, New Concerns*. Thousand Oaks, CA: SAGE Publications, 2003

Hughes, Alex, and Andrea Noble, editors. *Phototextualities: Intersections of Photography and Narrative*. Albuquerque: University of New Mexico Press, 2003

Hunt, Jennifer C. *Psychoanalytic Aspects of Fieldwork*. Newbury Park, CA: SAGE Publications, 1989

Hunter, Margaret L. *Race, Gender and the Politics of Skin Tone*. New York and London: Routledge, 2005

Hurst, Rachel Alpha Johnston. "Negotiating Femininity with and through Mother-Daughter and Patient-Surgeon Relationships in Cosmetic Surgery Narratives." *Women's Studies International Forum* 35, no. 6 (2012): 447–57

– "The Skin-Textile in Cosmetic Surgery." In *Skin, Culture and Psychoanalysis*, edited by Sheila L. Cavanagh, Angela Failler, and Rachel Alpha Johnston Hurst, 141–66. Houndsmills: Palgrave, 2013

– "Surgical Stories, Gendered Telling: Cosmetic Surgery through the Perspective of Patients and Surgeons." In *Gender Scripts in Medicine and Narrative*, edited by Marcelline Block and Angela Laflen, 269–90 Newcastle-Upon-Tyne: Cambridge Scholars Press, 2010

Huss-Ashmore, Rebecca. "'The Real Me': Therapeutic Narrative in Cosmetic Surgery." *Expedition* 42, no. 3 (2000): 26–37

Illouz, Eva. *Cold Intimacies: The Making of Emotional Capitalism*. London: Polity Press, 2007

Ince, Kate. *ORLAN: Millennial Female*. Oxford: Berg Publishers, 2001

Isaacs, Susan. "The Nature and Function of Fantasy." *International Journal of Psycho-Analysis* 29 (1948): 73–97

Izzo, Kim. "Afraid to Show Your Hand? You're not Alone. After Botox and Lid-lifts and Lipo, Women Are Examining Their Aging Paws Like so Many Lady Macbeths. And Help Is Just a Nip and Tuck – or a Fat Graft – Away." *Globe and Mail*, 12 March 2005, L1

Jeffreys, Sheila. *Beauty and Misogyny: Harmful Cultural Practices in the West*. London: Routledge, 2005

Jerslev, Anne. "The Mediated Body: Cosmetic Surgery in Television Drama, Reality Television and Fashion Photography." *Nordicom Review* 27, no. 2 (2006): 133–51

Jones, Meredith. "Makeover Culture's Dark Side: Breasts, Death, and Lolo Ferrari." *Body and Society* 14, no. 1 (2008b): 89–104

– *Skintight: An Anatomy of Cosmetic Surgery*. Oxford: Berg, 2008a

Jugenburg, Martin. "Dr Martin Jugenburg Reviews." http://toronto

surgery.ca/Toronto-Cosmetic-Surgery-Reviews.html. Accessed 16 February 2014

Kagan, Cara. "Diary of a Modern Facelift." *Harper's Bazaar* 3532 (March 2006): 292–3

Kazanjian, Dodie. "The Wrinkles We Keep: Now That Science Can Wipe Every Line off Your Face, Dodie Kazanjian Wonders if a Few Well-earned Markers of Age Might Make Her Look Better, not Worse." *Vogue* (August 2006): 196

Kosowski, T.R., C. McCarthy, P.L. Reavey, A.M. Scott, E.G. Wilkins, S.J. Cano, A.F. Klassen, N. Carr, P.G. Cordeiro, and A.L. Pusic. "A Systematic Review of Patient-Reported Outcome Measures after Facial Cosmetic Surgery and/or Nonsurgical Facial Rejuvenation." *Plastic & Reconstructive Surgery* 123, no. 6 (2009): 1819–27

Kvale, Steimar. "The Psychoanalytic Interview as Qualitative Research." *Qualitative Inquiry* 5, no. 1 (1999): 87–113

Lacan, Jacques. *The Four Fundamental Concepts of Psychoanalysis*, translated by Alan Sheridan and edited by Jacques-Alain Miller. New York: W.W. Norton and Company, 1998

– "The Mirror Stage as Formative of the Function of the 'I' as Revealed in the Psychoanalytic Experience." In *Écrits: A Selection*, translated by Alan Sheridan, 1–7. New York: Norton, 1977

– *The Seminar of Jacques Lacan, Book VII: The Ethics of Psychoanalysis*, translated by Dennis Porter and edited by Jacques-Alain Miller. New York: W.W. Norton, 1992

– *The Seminar of Jacques Lacan, Book III: The Psychoses, 1955–1956*, translated by Russell Grigg and edited by Jacques-Alain Miller. New York: W.W. Norton, 1993

Laliberté, Jennifer. "New Vaginas for Old: Cosmetic Surgery's Continuing Search for Lucrative New Frontiers." *National Review of Medicine* 3, no. 2 (January 2006). http://www.nationalreviewofmedicine.com/issue/2006/01_30/3_patients_practice01_2.html. Accessed 12 April 2015

Lather, Patti. *Getting Smart: Feminist Research and Pedagogy with/in the Postmodern*. New York: Routledge, 1991

Lee, Charles. "Asian Eyelid Surgery." http://www.asiancosmeticsurgery.com/procedures/asian-eyelid-surgery/. Accessed 23 June 2014

Lemma, Alessandra. "The Body One Has and the Body One Is: Understanding the Transsexual's Need to Be Seen." *International Journal of Psychonalysis* 94, no. 2 (2013): 277–92

– *Under the Skin: A Psychoanalytic Study of Body Modification*. New York: Routledge, 2010

Lloyd, Genevieve. *The Man of Reason: 'Male' and 'Female' in Western Philosophy*. London: Methuen, 1984

Lury, Celia. *Prosthetic Culture: Photography, Memory and Identity*. London and New York: Routledge, 1998

Mahoney, Jill. "Designer Vaginas: The Latest in Sex and Plastic Surgery." *Globe and Mail*, 13 August 2005, A1

Martin, Julie. "Suffering for Beauty." *Chatelaine* 72, 10 (October 1999): 53–4

Masson, Jeffrey Moussaieff, editor and translator. *The Complete Letters of Sigmund Freud to Wilhelm Fleiss, 1887–1904*. Cambridge, MA: Harvard University Press, 1985

Matlock, David L. "The Laser Vaginal Rejuvenation Institute of Los Angeles." http://www.drmatlock.com. Accessed 26 July 2007

McClintock, Anne. *Imperial Leather: Race, Gender and Sexuality in the Colonial Contest*. New York and London: Routledge, 1995

Meiners, Erica. "Inquiries into the Regulation of Disordered Bodies: Selected Sick and Twisted Ethnographic Fictions." PhD diss., Simon Fraser University, 1998

Menninger, Karl. "Polysurgery and Polysurgical Addiction." *Psychoanalytic Quarterly* 3 (1934): 173–99

Meyerowitz, Joanne. "Beyond the Feminine Mystique: A Reassessment of Postwar Mass Culture, 1946–1958." In *Not June Cleaver: Women and Gender in Postwar America, 1945–1960*, edited by Joanne Meyerowitz, 382–408. Philadelphia: Temple University Press, 1994

Minh-Ha, Trinh T. *Framer/Framed*. New York and London: Routledge, 1991

Morgan, Kathryn Pauly. "Women and the Knife: Cosmetic Surgery and the Colonization of Women's Bodies." *Hypatia* 6, no. 3 (1991): 25–53

Mulvey, Laura. "Visual Pleasure and Narrative Cinema." *Screen* 16, no. 3 (1975): 6–18

Nanomaterial Science Lab, National Chung Cheng University. "Skin Structure." http://www.nmsl.chem.ccu.edu.tw/tea/SKIN_910721.htm. Accessed 18 October 2007

Narayan, Kirin, and Kenneth M. George. "Personal and Folk Narrative as Cultural Representation." In Holstein and Gubrium, *Inside Interviewing*, 123–39

Naugler, Diane. "'To Take a Load Off': A Contextual Analysis of Gendered Meaning(s) in Experiences of Breast Reduction Surgery." PhD diss., York University, 2005

Northrop, Jane Megan. *Reflecting on Cosmetic Surgery: Body Image, Shame, and Narcissism*. London: Routledge, 2012

O'Bryan, Jill. *Carnal Art: ORLAN's Refacing*. Minneapolis: Minnesota University Press, 2005

Oliver, Kelly. *The Colonization of Psychic Space: A Psychoanalytic Social Theory of Oppression*. Minneapolis: University of Minnesota Press, 2004

Ontario Ministry of Health and Long-Term Care. "Schedule of Benefits for Physician Services under the Health Insurance Act, Appendix D: Surface

Pathology, Sub-Surface Pathology." http://www.health.gov.on.ca/english/
   providers/program/ohip/sob/physserv/append.pdf. Accessed 20 June 2014
ORLAN. Personal website. http://www.orlan.net. Accessed 21 October 2008
– "The Future of the Body with Performance Artist ORLAN." YouTube
   video, 1:24:27, posted by "Science Gallery Dublin," 1 July 2014.
   http://youtu.be/PjxEWPAnxDc. Accessed 5 February 2015
Ouellette, Laurie, and James Hay. *Better Living through Reality TV: Televi-
   sion and Post-Welfare Citizenship.* Malden, MA: Blackwell, 2008
Phelan, Peggy. "Cinematic Skin." In *ORLAN: Le récit/The narrative*, edited
   by Marie Galey and Emily Ligniti, 70–9. Milan: Charta, 2007
Pitts, Victoria. *In the Flesh: The Cultural Politics of Body Modification.*
   New York: Palgrave, 2003
Prosser, Jay. *Light in the Dark Room: Photography and Loss.* Minneapolis:
   Minnesota University Press, 2005
– *Second Skins: The Body Narratives of Transsexuality.* New York: Colum-
   bia University Press, 1998
Rapport, Frances. "The Poetry of Holocaust Survivor Testimony: Toward a
   New Performative Social Science." *Forum Qualitative Sozialforschung/
   Forum: Qualitative Social Research* 9, no. 2 (2008), Art. 28, http://nbn-
   resolving.de/urn:nbn:de:0114-fqs0802285. Accessed 13 July 2008
Richardson, Laurel. "Poetic Representations of Interviews." In Holstein
   and Gubrium, *Handbook of Interview Research*, 877–91
Rogers, Blair O. "The First Pre- and Post-Operative Photographs of Plastic
   and Reconstructive Surgery: Contributions of Gurdon Buck (1807–
   1877)." *Aesthetic Plastic Surgery* 15 (1991): 19–33
Rogers, Blair O., and Michael G. Rhond. "The First Civil War Photographs of Soldiers with Facial Wounds." *Aesthetic Plastic Surgery* 19
   (1995): 269–83
Roseneil, Sasha. "The Ambivalences of Angel's 'Arrangement'": A Psychosocial Lens on the Contemporary Condition of Personal Life." *Sociological
   Review* 54, no. 4 (2006): 847–69
Salecl, Renata. "Cut in the Body: From Clitoridectomy to Body Art." In
   Thinking through the Skin, edited by Sara Ahmed and Jackie Stacey,
   21–35. New York: Routledge, 2001
Sarwer, D.B., A.L. Infield, J.L. Baker, L.A. Casas, P.M. Glat, A.H. Gold,
   M.L. Jewell, D. LaRossa, F. Nahai, and V.L. Young. "Two-Year Results
   of a Prospective, Multi-Site Investigation of Patient Satisfaction and Psy-
   chosocial Status Following Cosmetic Surgery." *Aesthetic Surgery Journal*
   28, no. 3 (2008): 245–50
Scarry, Elaine. *The Body in Pain: The Making and Unmaking of the World.*
   New York and Oxford: Oxford University Press, 1985
Schilder, Paul. *The Image and Appearance of the Human Body: Studies in
   the Constructive Energies of the Psyche.* New York: International Univer-
   sities Press, 1950

Seshadri-Crooks, Kalpana. *Desiring Whiteness: A Lacanian Analysis of Race*. New York and London: Routledge, 2000

Shostak, John. *Interviewing and Representation in Qualitative Research*. New York: Open University Press, 2006

Siegel, Elizabeth. "Talking through the 'Fotygraft Album.'" In Hughes and Noble, *Phototextualities*, 239–53

Silverman, Kaja. *The Threshold of the Visible World*. New York and London: Routledge, 1996

Sobchack, Vivian. "Scary Women: Cinema, Surgery, and Special Effects." In Heyes and Jones, *Cosmetic Surgery: A Feminist Primer*, 79–95

Sontag, Susan. *On Photography*. New York: Picador, 1973

Spelman, Elizabeth. "Woman as Body: Ancient and Contemporary Views." *Feminist Studies* 8, no. 1 (1982): 109–31

Spitzack, Carole. "The Confession Mirror: Plastic Images for Surgery." *Canadian Journal of Social and Political Theory* 12, no. 1/2 (1988): 38–50

Stacey, Michelle. "Are Butts the New Boobs?" *Cosmopolitan* 241, 2 (August 2006): 154–7

Stepansky, Paul E. *Freud, Surgery, and the Surgeons*. Hillsdale, NJ: Analytic Press, 1999

Sullivan, Deborah A. *Cosmetic Surgery: The Cutting Edge of Commercial Medicine in America*. New Brunswick, NJ: Rutgers University Press, 2001

Sullivan, Nikki. "The Role of Medicine in the (Trans)Formation of 'Wrong' Bodies." *Body & Society* 14, no. 1 (2008): 105–16

Thomas, Mary E. "The Implications of Psychoanalysis for Qualitative Methodology: The Case of Interviews and Narrative Data Analysis." *The Professional Geographer* 54, no. 4 (2007): 537–46

Van Pelt, Tamise. *The Other Side of Desire*. Albany: State University of New York Press, 2000

Von Soest, T., I.L. Kvalem, H.E. Roald, and K.C. Skolleborg. "The Effects of Cosmetic Surgery on Body Image, Self-Esteem, and Psychological Problems." *Journal of Plastic, Reconstructive & Aesthetic Surgery* 62, no. 10 (2007): 1238–44

Von Soest, T., I.L. Kvalem, K.C. Skolleborg, and H.E. Roald. "Psychosocial Changes after Cosmetic Surgery: A 5-Year Follow-Up Study." *Plastic & Reconstructive Surgery* 128, no. 3 (2011): 765–72

Wegenstein, Bernadette. *The Cosmetic Gaze: Body Modification and the Construction of Beauty*. Cambridge: MIT Press, 2012

Williams, Mary E., editor. *Self-Mutilation*. Detroit: Greenhaven Press, 2008

Wong, Jan. "A Closer Look at the Double-fold Dream." *Globe and Mail*, 29 January 2005, M3

Yeo, Ji. Personal website. http://www.jiyeo.com. Accessed 13 February 2015

Žižek, Slavoj. *Looking Awry: An Introduction to Jacques Lacan through Popular Culture*. Cambridge: MIT Press, 1992

Zong, Oliver. "The Pinky Toe Tuck." http://www.readbag.com/nycfoot
  care-media-media-docs-skindeep. Accessed 11 April 2015
Zong, Oliver, and Dina Tsentserensky. "NYCFootcare." http://www.nyc
  footcare.com Accessed 24 July 2007

INDEX

Page numbers followed by "f" refer to figures. Page numbers followed by "n" refer to notes and are followed by the note number.